# Lecture Notes:
# **Dermatology**

## Robin Graham-Brown

BSc (Hons) (Lond), MB BS (Lond), FRCP, FRCPCH
Consultant Dermatologist
University Hospitals of Leicester
Honorary Senior Lecturer in Dermatology
University of Leicester

## Tony Burns

MB BS (Hons) (Lond), FRCP
Emeritus Consultant Dermatologist
The Leicester Royal Infirmary, Leicester

Tenth Edition

**WILEY-BLACKWELL**
A John Wiley & Sons, Ltd., Publication

*Library of Congress Cataloging-in-Publication Data*

Graham-Brown, R. A. C. (Robin A. C.)
    Lecture notes. Dermatology / Robin Graham-Brown, Tony Burns. – 10th ed.
        p. ; cm.
    Other title: Dermatology
    Includes bibliographical references and index.
    ISBN 978-1-4051-9571-3 (pbk.:alk. paper)   1. Dermatology–Outlines, syllabi, etc.
2. Skin–Diseases–Outlines, syllabi, etc.   I. Burns, Tony, FRCP.   II. Title.   III. Title:
Dermatology.
    [DNLM: 1.  Skin Diseases. WR 140]
    RL74.3.G73 2011
    616.5–dc22
                              2010031868

ISBN: 9781405195713

A catalogue record for this book is available from the British Library.

Set in 8.5 on 11 pt Utopia by Toppan Best-set Premedia Limited
Printed and bound in Singapore by Markono Print Media Pte Ltd

1   2011

Lecture N

**Dermat**

# Contents

# Contributor

*Chapter 23: Dermatological emergencies*

**Matthew Graham-Brown**
BSc (Hons) (Birmingham),
MB ChB (Hons) (Leicester Warwick)
Foundation Year 2
West Midlands Deanery

# Preface

In this, the tenth edition of *Lecture Notes: Dermatology*, we have updated the text, focusing on recent advances in the knowledge of skin diseases and their treatment. We have also asked a junior doctor working in an acute hospital in the UK to help us add a new chapter on dermatological emergencies.

Numerous tables of salient points provide ready reference but, as in previous editions, we have attempted to create a 'user-friendly' readability.

We hope that the book will be of value not only to medical students, but also to general practitioners, and nurses involved in the care of dermatology patients. We also hope that exposure to *Lecture Notes: Dermatology* will stimulate a deeper interest in this important medical specialty.

*Robin Graham-Brown*
*Tony Burns*

# Acknowledgements

We are indebted to the late Dr Imrich Sarkany, and to Professor Charles Calnan, under whose guidance we both learned dermatology.

We thank our colleagues in the Dermatology Department in Leicester: Drs Anton Alexandroff, Ian Anderson and Robert Burd, Professor Richard Camp and Drs Karen Harman, Ingrid Helbling, Peter Hutchinson, Graham Johnston, Alex Milligan, Joy Osborne and numerous junior colleagues for creating and sustaining such a stimulating environment in which to work.

It is a pleasure to have been joined for this edition by Matthew Graham-Brown, who has provided an excellent chapter on dermatological emergencies, for which we thank him very much.

We are especially grateful to all the medical students who, over many years, have reminded us of the importance of clarity in communication, and that teaching should be a stimulating and enjoyable experience for everyone concerned.

Finally, we thank the staff at Wiley-Blackwell who have helped us through the editing and production stages.

# Structure and function of the skin, hair and nails

*Skin, skin is a wonderful thing,*
*Keeps the outside out and the inside in.*

It is essential to have some background knowledge of the normal structure and function of any organ before you can hope to understand the abnormal. Skin is the icing on the anatomical cake, it is the decorative wrapping paper, and without it not only would we all look rather unappealing, but also a variety of unpleasant physiological phenomena would bring about our demise. You have probably never contemplated your skin a great deal, except in the throes of narcissistic admiration, or when it has been blemished by some disorder, but hopefully by the end of this first chapter you will have been persuaded that it is quite a remarkable organ, and that you are lucky to be on such intimate terms with it.

## Skin structure

The skin is composed of two layers, the epidermis and the dermis (Figure 1.1). The epidermis, which is the outer layer, and its appendages (hair, nails, sebaceous glands and sweat glands), are derived from the embryonic ectoderm. The dermis is of mesodermal origin.

*Lecture Notes: Dermatology*, 10th edition. © RAC Graham-Brown and DA Burns. Published 2011 by Blackwell Publishing Ltd.

## The epidermis

The epidermis is a stratified squamous epithelium, with several well-defined layers. The principal cell type is known as a *keratinocyte*. Keratinocytes, produced by cell division in the deepest layer of the epidermis (basal layer), are carried towards the skin surface, undergoing in transit a complex series of morphological and biochemical changes known as *terminal differentiation* (keratinization) to produce the surface layer of tightly packed dead cells (stratum corneum or horny layer) which are eventually shed. In health the rate of production of cells matches the rate of loss so that epidermal thickness is constant. Epidermal kinetics are controlled by a number of growth stimulators and inhibitors.

The components of this differentiation process are under genetic control and mutations in the controlling genes are responsible for a variety of diseases.

So-called *intermediate filaments*, present in the cytoplasm of epithelial cells, are a major component of the cytoskeleton. They contain a group of fibrous proteins known as keratins, each of which is the product of a separate gene. Pairs of keratins are characteristic of certain cell types and tissues. The mitotically active keratinocytes in the basal layer express the keratin pair K5/K14, but during the differentiation process expression of K5/K14 is down-regulated and that of K1/K10 is induced.

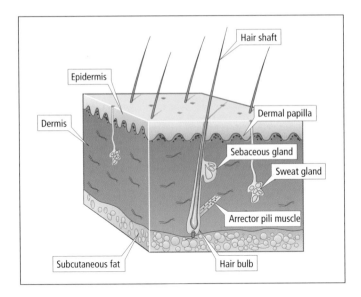

Figure 1.1 The structure of the skin.

As cells reach the higher layers of the epidermis, keratin filaments aggregate into keratin fibrils under the influence of a protein known as *filaggrin* (filament-aggregating protein)—this is derived from its precursor *profilaggrin*, present in *keratohyalin granules* which constitute the granules in the granular layer. Derivatives of the proteolysis of filaggrin are major components of natural moisturizing factor (NMF) which is important in the maintenance of epidermal hydration. Loss-of-function mutations in *FLG*, the gene encoding filaggrin, underlie ichthyosis vulgaris and strongly predispose to atopic eczema; carriers of these mutations have reduced levels of NMF in the stratum corneum.

In the final stages of terminal differentiation, the plasma membrane is replaced by the *cornified cell envelope*, composed of several proteins the production of which is also under genetic control. Cells that have developed this envelope and have lost their nucleus and organelles constitute the *corneocytes* of the stratum corneum.

Look at the layers more closely (Figure 1.2). The basal layer, which is one to three cells thick, is anchored to a basement membrane (see below) that lies between the epidermis and dermis. Interspersed among the basal cells are melanocytes—large dendritic cells derived from the neural crest—that are responsible for melanin pigment production. Melanocytes contain cytoplasmic organelles called melanosomes, in which melanin is synthesized from tyrosine. The melanosomes

migrate along the dendrites of the melanocytes and are transferred to the keratinocytes in the prickle cell layer. In white people the melanosomes are grouped together in membrane-bound *melanosome complexes*, and they gradually degenerate as the keratinocytes move towards the surface of the skin. The skin of black people contains the same number of melanocytes as that of white people, but the melanosomes are larger, remain separate and persist through the full thickness of the epidermis. The main stimulus to melanin production is ultraviolet (UV) radiation. Melanin protects the cell nuclei in the epidermis from the harmful effects of UV radiation. A suntan is a natural protective mechanism, not some God-given cosmetic boon created so that you can impress the neighbours on your return from an exotic foreign trip! Unfortunately, this does not appear to be appreciated by the pale, pimply, lager-swilling advert for British manhood who dashes onto the beach in Ibiza and flash fries himself to lobster thermidor on day one of his annual holiday.

Skin neoplasia is extremely uncommon in dark-skinned races because their skin is protected from UV damage by the large amounts of melanin that it contains. However, individuals with albinism are predisposed to skin cancer because their production of melanin is impaired and they are therefore without its protective influence.

Above the basal layer is the prickle cell/spinous layer. This acquires its name from the

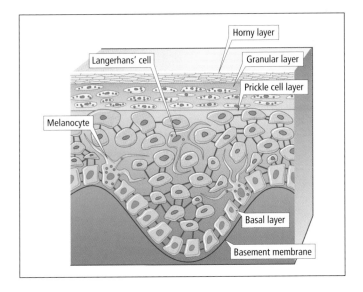

Figure 1.2 The epidermis.

spiky appearance produced by the intercellular bridges (desmosomes) that connect adjacent cells. Important in cell–cell adhesion are several protein components of desmosomes (including cadherins [desmogleins and desmocollins] and plakins). Production of these is genetically controlled, and abnormalities have been detected in some human diseases.

Scattered throughout the prickle cell layer are Langerhans' cells. These dendritic cells contain characteristic racquet-shaped 'Birbeck' granules. Langerhans' cells are probably modified macrophages, which originate in the bone marrow and migrate to the epidermis. They are the first line of immunological defence against environmental antigens (see below).

Above the prickle cell layer is the granular layer, which is composed of flattened cells containing the darkly staining keratohyalin granules. Also present in the cytoplasm of cells in the granular layer are organelles known as lamellar granules (Odland bodies). These contain lipids and enzymes, and they discharge their contents into the intercellular spaces between the cells of the granular layer and stratum corneum—providing the equivalent of 'mortar' between the cellular 'bricks', and contributing to the barrier function of the epidermis.

The cells of the stratum corneum are flattened, keratinized cells that are devoid of nuclei and cytoplasmic organelles. Adjacent cells overlap at their margins, and this locking together of cells, together with intercellular lipid, forms a very effective barrier. The stratum corneum varies in thickness according to the region of the body. It is thickest on the palms of the hands and soles of the feet. The stratum corneum cells are gradually abraded by daily wear and tear. If you bathe after a period of several days' avoidance of water (a house without central heating, in mid-winter, somewhere in the Northern Hemisphere, is ideal for this experiment), you will note that as you towel yourself you are rubbing off small balls of keratin—which has built up because of your unsanitary habits. When a plaster cast is removed from a fractured limb after several weeks *in situ* there is usually a thick layer of surface keratin, the removal of which provides hours of absorbing occupational therapy.

Figure 1.3 shows the histological appearance of normal epidermis.

## The basement membrane zone

This is composed of a number of layers, and it is important to have some knowledge of these because certain diseases are related to abnormalities in the layers. The basic structure is shown in Figure 1.4. Basal keratinocytes are attached by *hemidesmosomes* to the epidermal side of the membrane, and these have an important role in maintaining adhesion between the epidermis and dermis. The basement membrane is composed of three layers: lamina lucida (uppermost), lamina densa and lamina fibroreticularis. A system of *anchoring filaments* connects hemidesmosomes to the lamina densa, and *anchoring fibrils*, which are closely associated with collagen in the upper dermis, connect the lamina densa to the dermis beneath.

The hemidesmosome/anchoring filament region contains autoantigens targeted by autoantibodies in immunobullous disorders (including bullous pemphigoid, pemphigoid gestationis, cicatricial pemphigoid and linear IgA bullous dermatosis—see Chapter 14), hence the subepidermal location of blistering in these disorders.

The inherited blistering diseases (see Chapter 14) occur as a consequence of mutations in genes responsible for components of the basement membrane zone, e.g. epidermolysis bullosa simplex, in which splits occur in the basal keratinocytes, is related to mutations in genes coding for keratins 5 and 14, and dystrophic epidermolysis bullosa, in which blistering occurs immediately below the lamina densa, is related to mutations in a gene coding for type VII collagen, the major component of anchoring fibrils.

## Epidermal appendages

The eccrine and apocrine sweat glands, the hair and sebaceous glands, and the nails, constitute the epidermal appendages.

### Eccrine sweat glands

Eccrine sweat glands are important in body temperature regulation. A human has between two and three million eccrine sweat glands covering almost all the body surface. They are particularly numerous on the palms of the hands and soles of the feet. Each consists of a secretory coil deep in the dermis, and a duct that conveys the sweat to the surface. Eccrine glands secrete water, electrolytes, lactate, urea and ammonia. The secretory coil produces isotonic sweat, but sodium chloride is reabsorbed in the duct so that sweat reaching the surface is hypotonic. Patients with cystic fibrosis have defective reabsorption of sodium chloride, and rapidly become salt depleted in a hot environment. Eccrine sweat glands are innervated

**Figure 1.3** Section of skin stained with haematoxylin and eosin, showing the appearance of a normal epidermis. 'Rete ridges' (downward projections of the epidermis) interdigitate with 'dermal papillae' (upward projections of the dermis).

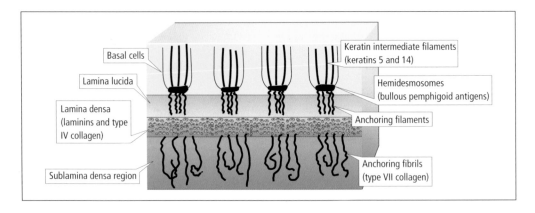

**Figure 1.4** Structure of the basement membrane zone.

by the sympathetic nervous system, but the neurotransmitter is acetylcholine.

## Apocrine sweat glands

Apocrine sweat glands are found principally in the axillae and anogenital region. Specialized apocrine glands include the wax glands of the ear and the milk glands of the breast. Apocrine glands are also composed of a secretory coil and a duct, but the duct opens into a hair follicle, not directly on to the surface of the skin. Apocrine glands produce an oily secretion containing protein, carbohydrate, ammonia and lipid. These glands become active at puberty, and secretion is controlled by adrenergic nerve fibres. Pungent axillary body odour (axillary bromhidrosis) is the result of the action of bacteria on apocrine secretions. In some animals apocrine secretions are important sexual attractants, but the average human armpit provides a different type of overwhelming olfactory experience.

## Hair

Hairs grow out of tubular invaginations of the epidermis known as follicles, and a hair follicle and its associated sebaceous glands are referred to as a 'pilosebaceous unit'. There are three types of hair: fine, soft *lanugo* hair is present *in utero* and is shed by the eighth month of fetal life; *vellus* hair is the fine downy hair that covers most of the body except those areas occupied by terminal hair; and thick and pigmented *terminal* hair occurs on the scalp, eyebrows and eyelashes before puberty—after puberty, under the influence of androgens, secondary sexual terminal hair develops from vellus hair in the axillae and pubic region, and on the trunk and limbs in men. On the scalp, the reverse occurs in male-pattern balding—terminal hair becomes vellus hair under the influence of androgens. In men, terminal hair on the body usually increases in amount as middle age arrives, and hairy ears and nostrils, and bushy eyebrows, are puzzling accompaniments of advancing years. One struggles to think of any biological advantage conferred by exuberant growth of hair in these sites.

Hair follicles extend into the dermis at an angle (see Figure 1.1). A small bundle of smooth muscle fibres, the arrector pili muscle, is attached to the side of the follicle. Arrector pili muscles are supplied by adrenergic nerves, and are responsible for the erection of hairs in the cold or during emotional stress ('goose flesh', 'goose pimples', horripilation). The duct of the sebaceous gland enters the follicle just above the point of attachment of the arrector pili muscle. At the lower end of the follicle is the hair bulb, part of which, the hair matrix, is a zone of rapidly dividing cells that is responsible for the formation of the hair shaft. Hair pigment is produced by melanocytes in the hair bulb. Cells produced in the hair bulb become densely packed, elongated and arranged parallel to the long axis of the hair shaft. They gradually become keratinized as they ascend in the hair follicle.

The main part of each hair fibre is the cortex, which is composed of keratinized spindle-shaped cells (Figure 1.5). Terminal hairs have a central core known as the medulla, consisting of specialized cells that contain air spaces. Covering the cortex is the cuticle, a thin layer of cells that overlap like the tiles on a roof, with the free margins of the cells pointing towards the tip of the hair. The cross-sectional shape of hair varies with body site and race. Negroid hair is distinctly oval in cross-section, and pubic, beard and eyelash hairs have an oval cross-section in all racial types. Caucasoid hair is moderately elliptical in cross-section and mongoloid hair is circular.

The growth of each hair is cyclical—periods of active growth alternate with resting phases. After each period of active growth (anagen) there is a short transitional phase (catagen), followed by a resting phase (telogen), after which the follicle reactivates, a new hair is produced and the old hair is shed. The duration of these cyclical phases depends on the age of the individual and the location of the follicle on the body. The duration of

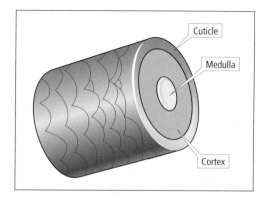

Figure 1.5 The structure of hair.

anagen in a scalp follicle is genetically determined, and ranges from 2 to more than 5 years. This is why some women can grow hair down to their ankles, whereas most have a much shorter maximum length. Scalp hair catagen lasts about 2 weeks and telogen from 3 months to 4 months. The daily growth rate of scalp hair is approximately 0.45 mm. The activity of each follicle is independent of that of its neighbours, which is fortunate, because, if follicular activity were synchronized, as it is in some animals, we would be subject to periodic moults, thus adding another dimension to life's rich tapestry. At any one time approximately 85% of scalp hairs are in anagen, 1% in catagen and 14% in telogen. The average number of hairs shed daily is 100. In areas other than the scalp anagen is relatively short—this is also fortunate, because, if it were not so, we would all be kept busy clipping eyebrows, eyelashes and nether regions.

It is a myth that shaving increases the rate of growth of hair and that it encourages the development of 'thicker' hair; nor does hair continue growing after death—shrinkage of soft tissues around the hair produces this illusion.

Human hair colour is principally dependent on two types of melanin: eumelanins in black and brown hair, and phaeomelanins in red, auburn and blond hair.

Greying of hair (canities) is the result of a decrease in tyrosinase activity in the melanocytes of the hair bulb. The age of onset of greying is genetically determined, but other factors may be involved such as autoimmunity—premature greying of the hair is a recognized association of pernicious anaemia. The phenomenon of 'going white overnight' has been attributed to severe psychological stress—it is said that the hair of Thomas Moore and Marie Antoinette turned white on the night before their executions. However, this is physically impossible unless related to the washing out of temporary hair dye, but it might occur over a period of a few days or weeks as a result of alopecia areata occurring in an individual with a mixture of white and pigmented hair in whom there was selective loss of pigmented hair.

## Sebaceous glands

Sebaceous glands are found everywhere on the skin apart from the hands and feet. They are particularly numerous and prominent on the head and neck, the chest and the back. Sebaceous glands are part of the pilosebaceous unit, and their lipid-rich product (sebum) flows through a duct into the hair follicle. They are holocrine glands—sebum is produced by disintegration of glandular cells rather than an active secretory process. Modified sebaceous glands that open directly on the surface are found on the eyelids, lips, nipples, glans penis and prepuce, and the buccal mucosa (Fordyce spots).

Sebaceous glands are prominent at birth, under the influence of maternal hormones, but atrophy soon after, and do not enlarge again until puberty. Enlargement of the glands and sebum production at puberty are stimulated by androgens. Growth hormone and thyroid hormones also affect sebum production.

## Nails

A nail is a transparent plate of keratin derived from an invagination of epidermis on the dorsum of the terminal phalanx of a digit (Figure 1.6). The nail plate is the product of cell division in the nail matrix, which lies deep to the proximal nail fold, but is partly visible as the pale 'half-moon' (lunula) at the base of the nail. The nail plate adheres firmly to the underlying nail bed. The cuticle is an extension of the horny layer of the proximal nail fold on to the nail plate. It forms a seal between

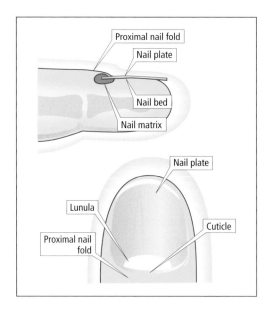

Figure 1.6 The nail.

the nail plate and proximal nail fold, preventing penetration of extraneous material.

Nail growth is continuous throughout life, but is more rapid in youth than in old age. The average rate of growth of fingernails is approximately 1 mm/week, and the time taken for a fingernail to grow from matrix to free edge is about 6 months. Nails on the dominant hand grow slightly more rapidly than those on the non-dominant hand. Toenails grow at one-third the rate of fingernails, and take about 18 months to grow from matrix to free edge.

Many factors affect nail growth rate. It is increased in psoriasis, and may be speeded up in the presence of inflammatory change around the nail. A severe systemic upset can produce a sudden slowing of nail growth, causing a transverse groove in each nail plate. These grooves, known as Beau's lines, subsequently become visible as the nails grow out. Nail growth may also be considerably slowed in the digits of a limb immobilized in plaster.

## The dermis

The dermis is a layer of connective tissue lying beneath the epidermis, and forms the bulk of the skin. The dermis and epidermis interdigitate via downward epidermal projections (rete ridges) and upward dermal projections (dermal papillae) (see Figures 1.1 and 1.3). The main feature of the dermis is a network of interlacing fibres, mostly collagen, but with some elastin. These fibres give the dermis great strength and elasticity. The collagen and elastin fibres, which are protein, are embedded in a ground substance of mucopolysaccharides (glycosaminoglycans).

The main cellular elements of the dermis are fibroblasts, mast cells and macrophages. Fibroblasts synthesize the connective tissue matrix of the dermis, and are usually found in close proximity to collagen and elastin fibres. Mast cells are specialized secretory cells present throughout the dermis, but they are more numerous around blood vessels and appendages. They contain granules the contents of which include mediators such as histamine, prostaglandins, leukotrienes, and eosinophil and neutrophil chemotactic factors. Macrophages are phagocytic cells that originate in the bone marrow, and they act as scavengers of cell debris and extracellular material. The dermis is also richly supplied with blood vessels, lymphatics, nerves and sensory receptors. Beneath the dermis, a layer of subcutaneous fat separates the skin from underlying fascia and muscle.

## Dermatoglyphics

Fingerprints, the characteristic elevated ridge patterns on the fingertips of humans, are unique to each individual. The fingers and toes, and the palms and soles, are covered with a system of ridges that form patterns. The term 'dermatoglyphics' is applied to the configuration of the ridges. If you look closely at your hands you will see these tiny ridges, which are separate from the skin creases. On the tips of the fingers there are three basic patterns: arches, loops and whorls (Figure 1.7). The loops are subdivided into ulnar or radial, depending on whether the loop is open to the ulnar or radial side of the hand. A triangular intersection of these ridges is known as a triradius, and these triradii are present not only on fingertips, but also at the base of each finger, and usually on the proximal part of the palm.

Not only are the ridge patterns of fingerprints useful for the identification and conviction of those who covet their neighbours' goods, but characteristic dermatoglyphic abnormalities frequently accompany many chromosomal aberrations.

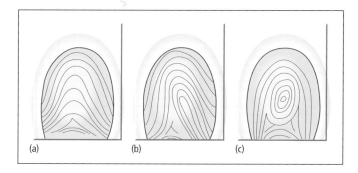

(a)  (b)  (c)

Figure 1.7 Dermatoglyphics: (a) arch; (b) loop; (c) whorl.

# Functions of the skin

*Skin is like wax paper that holds everything in without dripping.*

> Art Linkletter, A Child's Garden of
> Misinformation, 1965

It is obvious from the complex structure of the skin that it is not there simply to hold all the other bits of the body together. Some of the functions of skin are as shown in the box.

---

**Skin functions**

- Prevents loss of essential body fluids
- Protects against entry of toxic environmental chemicals and microorganisms
- Immunological functions
- Protects against damage from UV radiation
- Regulates body temperature
- Synthesis of vitamin D
- Important in sexual attraction and social interaction

---

In the absence of a stratum corneum we would lose significant amounts of water to the environment, and rapidly become dehydrated. The stratum corneum, with its overlapping cells and intercellular lipid, blocks diffusion of water into the environment. If it is removed by stripping with tape, water loss to the environment increases 10-fold or more.

It is also quite an effective barrier to the penetration of external agents. However, this barrier capacity is considerably reduced if the stratum corneum is hydrated, or its lipid content is reduced by the use of lipid solvents. The structural integrity of the stratum corneum also protects against invasion by microorganisms, and when there is skin loss, e.g. in burns or toxic epidermal necrolysis, infection is a major problem. Other factors, such as the acid pH of sweat and sebaceous secretions, antimicrobial peptides (AMPs), known as *defensins* and *cathelcidins*, that kill a variety of microbes, and complement components all contribute to antibacterial activity. The rarity of fungal infection of the scalp in adults is thought to be related to changes at puberty in the fatty acid composition of sebum, its constituents after puberty having fungistatic activity.

The skin is an immunologically competent organ and plays an important part in host defence against 'foreign' material. The dendritic Langerhans' cells are antigen-presenting cells that take up antigens, process them, and migrate to regional lymph nodes where the antigens, in association with major histocompatibility (MHC) class II, are presented to receptors on T cells. A naïve T cell that interacts with an antigen proliferates to form a clone that will recognize the antigen if re-exposed to it. Such primed (memory) T cells circulate around the body. If the antigen is encountered again the primed T cells are activated, and secrete cytokines that cause lymphocytes, polymorphonuclear leucocytes and monocytes to move into the area, thereby causing inflammation. This mechanism also forms the basis of the inflammatory reaction in allergic contact dermatitis.

Cytokines are polypeptides and glycoproteins secreted by cells (e.g. lymphocytes, macrophages and keratinocytes). They include interleukins, interferons (INFs), tumour necrosis factor (TNF), colony-stimulating factors and growth factors. Their main role is to regulate inflammatory and immune responses.

Although detailed discussion of immunology and inflammation is beyond the scope of this book it is important for you to understand some of the basic mechanisms involved for a variety of reasons, not least because such knowledge is necessary in order to comprehend the modes of action of the increasingly sophisticated treatments being developed, e.g. biological therapies, which are being used to treat psoriasis (see Chapter 8) by targeting components of its pathomechanism (see Chapter 22).

The protective effect of melanin against UV damage has already been mentioned, but in addition to this there is an important system of enzymes responsible for repair of UV-damaged DNA. Such damage occurs continuously and the consequences of a non-functioning repair system can be seen in the recessively inherited disorder xeroderma pigmentosum (XP). In XP, cumulative UV damage leads to development of skin neoplasia in childhood.

The skin is a vital part of the body's temperature regulation system. The body core temperature is regulated by a temperature-sensitive area in the hypothalamus, and this is influenced by the temperature of the blood that perfuses it. The response of the skin to cold is vasoconstriction and a marked reduction in blood flow, decreasing transfer of heat to the body surface. The response to heat is vasodilatation, an increase in skin blood flow and loss of heat to the environment. Perspiration helps to cool the body by evaporation of sweat. These thermoregulatory functions are impaired in certain skin diseases—patients with exfoliative dermatitis (erythroderma) radiate heat to their environment because their skin blood flow is considerably increased and they are unable to control this by vasoconstriction. In a cold environment their central core temperature drops, in spite of producing metabolic heat by shivering, and they may die of hypothermia.

Vitamin D (cholecalciferol) is produced in the skin by the action of UV light on dehydrocho-lesterol. In those whose diets are deficient in vitamin D this extra source of the vitamin can be important.

The skin is also a huge sensory receptor, perceiving heat, cold, pain, light touch and pressure, and even tickle. As you are probably still grappling with the conundrum of the biological significance of hairy ears in elderly men, try switching your thoughts to the benefits of tickly armpits!

In addition to all these mechanistic functions, the skin plays an essential aesthetic role in social interaction and sexual attraction.

Hence, you can see that your skin is doing a good job. Apart from looking pleasant, it is saving you from becoming a cold, UV-damaged, brittle-boned, desiccated 'prune'.

# 2

# Approach to the diagnosis of dermatological disease

*Baglivi has said, 'The patient is the doctor's best text-book'. That 'text-book', however, has to be introduced to the student and those who effect the introductions are not always wise.*
          *Dannie Abse,* Doctors and Patients

*The dermatologist's art is giving a disease a long Greek name ... and then a topical steroid.*
                                    *Anon*

## Introduction

Dermatology is essentially a specialty where clinical information is at the forefront of the diagnostic process, and it is important for any aspiring clinician to realize that, before prescribing treatment or offering prognostic information about a patient's problem, he or she must first make a diagnosis. This chapter is about reaching a diagnosis in a patient with a skin disorder.

### The value of a diagnosis

The facts on which a clinician makes a diagnosis *must* always come first and foremost from the patient, and there is no substitute for talking to

*Lecture Notes: Dermatology*, 10th edition. © RAC Graham-Brown and DA Burns. Published 2011 by Blackwell Publishing Ltd.

and examining patients. This is especially true of skin disease.

A diagnosis is a short statement about a disease state or condition.

---

**Diagnosis**

- Provides a working label that will be recognized by others
- Implies some commonality with other patients with the same disease state or condition: in aetiology; pathology; clinical features; responsiveness to treatment
- Offers a prognosis and information about contagion or heredity
- Gives access to treatment modalities

---

## Dermatological diagnosis

*That which we call a rose,*
*by any other name would smell as sweet*
                  *Shakespeare,* Romeo and Juliet

Aspiring dermatologists must begin by becoming familiar with the diagnostic labels used in the description and classification of skin disease. This can seem daunting, but remember that diagnostic labels in medicine are bound by convention and rooted in history: the nomenclature of disease, and its signs and symptoms, has emerged from hundreds of years of classification and categorization. There is nothing special about dermatology, except perhaps in the degree to which subtle clinical variations are afforded separate names. The fact that diagnostic terms often bear no relationship to modern thinking is not of itself important. An apple is still an apple, even if we don't know who first called it that or why!

Therefore, as in any other branch of medicine, the diagnostic terminology in dermatology has to be learned. This may take time, but is not as hard as it may at first seem. In the same way that someone moving to a foreign country has to become used to a new vocabulary, the dermatological tyro who pays attention rapidly becomes acquainted with the more common skin changes and the diseases that cause them (e.g. eczema, psoriasis or warts). In time, he or she will also begin to recognize rarer disorders and less 'classic' variants of more common ones. However, this remains a dynamic process that involves seeing, reading, asking and learning—always with the eyes, ears and mind open!

## The steps to making a dermatological diagnosis

In principle, there is nothing more difficult about diagnosing diseases of the skin than those of any other organ. The process of identification consists of taking a history, examining the patient and performing investigations where necessary. In practice, many dermatologists will ask questions *after* a quick look to assess the problem, and also during the formal examination. However, we should consider the elements of the process separately.

A dermatological history contains most of the questions that you will be used to asking: onset and duration, fluctuation, exacerbating or ameliorating factors, nature of symptoms, past history. There are some differences, however, that are largely in the emphasis placed on certain aspects, shown above.

There are also specific features of dermatological histories to watch out for.

## Symptoms

Patients with skin disease talk about symptoms, especially itching, which you may not have met before. You will soon get used to assessing and quantifying these. For example, a severe itch will keep patients awake or stop them from concentrating at work or school.

## Patients' language

Be careful about terms that patients use to describe their skin problems. In Leicestershire, where the authors work, weals are often called 'blisters' and it is easy to be misled. Always ask the patient to describe precisely what he or she means by a specific term.

## Quality of life

It may be very helpful to assess the impact of the problem on the patient's normal daily activities and self-image: work, school, sleep, self-confidence, personal relationships. An understanding of the effect of skin disease on friends and family is important too.

---

### Dermatological history

**Past history**

Should include:

- General health problems, such as diabetes and TB
- Past skin problems
- Significant allergies or intolerances

**Family history**

- Some disorders are infectious; others have strong genetic backgrounds

**Occupation and hobbies**

- The skin is frequently affected by materials encountered at work and in the home

**Therapy**

- Not only *systemic* medication but also *topical* remedies; many patients apply multiple creams, lotions and ointments; topicals may be prescribed medicines, or self-administered, with or without advice from others (patients nearly always forget the names)

BUT

- *Topical applications* may also be part of a 'cosmetic' regimen

## Patient preconceptions

Patients often have their own ideas about the cause of skin problems and will readily offer them! For example, washing powder or detergent is almost universally considered to be a major cause of rashes, and injuries to be triggers of skin tumours. Never ignore what you are told, but take care to sieve the information in the light of your findings.

Watch out, too, for the very high expectations of many patients. They know that visible evidence is there for all to see: dermatology often truly requires a 'spot' diagnosis! Everyone from the patient and his or her relatives to the local green-grocer can see the problem and express their opinion (and usually have).

## Examination

The next step is to examine the patient. Wise counsels maintain that you should *always* examine a patient from head to foot. In reality this can be hard on both patient and doctor, especially if the problem is a solitary wart on the thumb! However, as a general rule, and especially with inflammatory dermatoses and conditions with several lesions, you should have an overall look at the sites

---

### Dermatological assessment

1 **Site(s) and/or distribution:** this can be very helpful, e.g. psoriasis has a predilection for knees, elbows, scalp and lower back; eczema favours the flexures in children; acne occurs predominantly on the face and upper trunk; basal cell carcinomas are more common on the head and neck

2 **Characteristics of individual lesion(s):**
   - **The type:** some simple preliminary reading is essential; use Table 2.1 for the most common and important terms and their definitions
   - **The size:** size is best *measured*, rather than being a comparison with peas, oranges or coins of the realm
   - **The shape:** lesions may be various shapes, e.g. round, oval, annular, linear or 'irregular'; straight edges and angles may suggest external factors
   - **The outline and border:** the outline is irregular in a superficial spreading melanoma, but smooth in most benign lesions; the border is well defined in psoriasis, but blurred in most patches of eczema
   - **The colour:** it is always useful to note the colour: red, purple, brown, slate-black, etc.
   - **Surface features** (Table 2.1): it is helpful to assess whether the surface is smooth or rough, and to distinguish crust (dried serum) from scale (hyperkeratosis); some assessment of scale can be helpful, e.g. 'silvery' in psoriasis
   - **The texture—superficial? deep?** Use your fingertips on the surface; assess the depth and position in or beneath the skin; lift scale or crust to see what is underneath; try to make the lesion blanch with pressure

3 **Secondary sites:** look for additional features that may assist in diagnosis. Good examples of this include:
   - The nails in psoriasis
   - The fingers and wrists in scabies
   - The toe webs in fungal infections
   - The mouth in lichen planus

4 **'Special' techniques:** these are covered in the appropriate chapters, but there are some tricks, e.g.
   - Scraping a psoriatic plaque for capillary bleeding
   - The Nikolsky sign in blistering diseases
   - 'Diascopy' in suspected cutaneous tuberculosis
   - 'Dermatoscopy', especially for pigmented lesions

It is fair to say that in inflammatory dermatoses a complication is having to decide *which lesion or lesions to select* for assessment and analysis. Skin diseases are dynamic. Some lesions in any rash will be very early, some very late and some at various intermediate evolutionary stages.

Try to examine as many patients as you can: frequent exposure to skin diseases helps you to develop an ability to recognize those lesions that provide the most useful diagnostic information.

The diagnostic process will gradually become one that you will perform increasingly easily and confidently as experience develops.

involved. You may also find the unexpected, such as melanomas and other skin cancers.

Inspect *and palpate* the lesion(s) or rash. It may help to use a magnifying hand lens or a dermatoscope, especially for pigmented lesions.

The fundamental elements of a good dermatological examination are:

1 Site and/or distribution of the problem
2 Characteristics of individual lesion(s)
3 Examination of 'secondary' sites
4 'Special' techniques

Unfortunately, names and terms can appear to get in the way of learning in dermatology. Indeed this is one reason why many clinicians claim that dermatology is a mysterious and impenetrable mixture of mumbo-jumbo and strange potions. There is really no need for this: the terms in use have developed for good reasons. They provide a degree of precision and a framework for diagnosis and decision-making. Try to familiarize yourself with them and apply them correctly. They will provide the building blocks to go on and make dermatological diagnoses more easily and more accurately. So, in the early days, describe everything that you see in these terms as far as possible.

## Investigation

Inevitably, history and examination alone will not always provide all the information required to produce a satisfactory working diagnosis. There are some skin disorders in which further investigation is nearly always necessary: to confirm a diagnosis with important prognostic or therapeutic implications (e.g. blistering disorders), to plan optimal management or to seek an underlying, associated systemic disorder (e.g. in generalized pruritus). These situations are covered later in the appropriate chapters. Advances in modern genetics, too, mean that blood (or other tissues) can be analysed for evidence of specific defects.

A number of important techniques are available that can provide further information. Some of these, such as appropriate blood tests and swabs for bacteriology and virology, should be familiar from other branches of medicine, and are fully covered in other introductory textbooks.

---

**Table 2.1 Types and characteristics of lesions (see Figure 2.1)**

### Lesion characteristics
- Macule: a flat, circumscribed area of skin discoloration
- Papule: a circumscribed elevation of the skin <0.5 cm in diameter
- Nodule: a circumscribed visible or palpable lump, >0.5 cm
- Plaque: a circumscribed, disc-shaped, elevated area of skin:
  'small'<2 cm in diameter
  'large'>2 cm in diameter
- Vesicle: a small visible collection of fluid (≤0.5 cm in diameter)
- Bulla: a large visible collection of fluid (≥0.5 cm)
- Pustule: a visible accumulation of pus
- Ulcer: a loss of epidermis (often with loss of underlying dermis and subcutis as well)
- Weal: a circumscribed, elevated area of cutaneous oedema

### Surface characteristics
- Scale: visible and palpable flakes due to aggregation and/or abnormalities of shed epidermal cells
- Crust: accumulated dried exudate, e.g. serum
- Horn: an elevated projection of keratin
- Excoriation: a secondary, superficial ulceration, due to scratching
- Maceration: an appearance of surface softening due to constant wetting
- Lichenification: a flat-topped thickening of the skin often secondary to scratching

Figure 2.1 Lesion characteristics: (a) macule (pityriasis versicolor); (b) papule (molluscum contagiosum); (c) nodule (nodular prurigo); (d) plaque (psoriasis); (e) vesicle (herpes zoster); (f) bulla (bullous insect bite reaction); (g) pustule; (h) ulcer (venous ulcer); (i) weal (urticaria/dermographism).

Others, however, are more specific to dermatological investigation. Useful tests include the following:

- Blood tests: for underlying systemic abnormalities and, increasingly, for genetic analysis
- Swabs and other samples: for infections
- Wood's light: some disorders/features are easier to see

- Skin scrapes or nail clippings: microscopy and mycological culture
- Skin biopsy: histopathology; electron microscopy; immunopathology; DNA phenotyping
- Prick tests: occasionally helpful in elucidating type I allergies (they have little or no place in the investigation of eczema)
- Patch tests: for evidence of contact allergy

Figure 2.1 *Continued*

## Wood's light

This is a nickel oxide-filtered UV light source, used to highlight three features of skin disease:

1 Certain organisms that cause scalp ringworm produce green fluorescence (useful in initial diagnosis and helpful in assessing therapy)
2 The organism responsible for erythrasma fluoresces coral-pink
3 Some pigmentary disorders are more clearly visible in this light—particularly the pale patches of tuberous sclerosis and café-au-lait marks of neurofibromatosis

Wood's light can also be used to induce fluorescence in the urine in some of the porphyrias.

## Scrapings/clippings

Material from the skin, hair or nails can be examined directly under the microscope and/or sent for culture. This is particularly useful in suspected fungal infection, or in a search for scabies mites (see Chapters 4 and 5). Scraping lightly at the epidermis will lift scales from the surface of the suspicious area.

The scales are placed on a microscope slide, covered with 10% potassium hydroxide (KOH) and a coverslip. After a few minutes to dissolve some of the epidermal cell membranes, they can be examined. It is helpful to add some Parker Quink ink if an infection with *Malassezia* (*Pityrosporum*) species (the cause of pityriasis versicolor) is

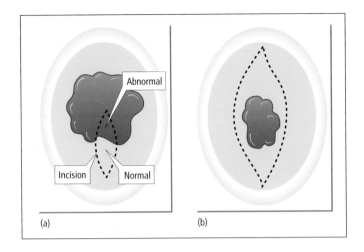

(a)                (b)

Figure 2.2 The technique for incisional (a) and (b) excisional biopsy.

suspected. Nail clippings can also be treated this way, but need stronger solutions of KOH or longer to dissolve.

Microscopy of hair may also provide information about fungal infections, reveal structural hair shaft abnormalities in certain genetic disorders and be useful in distinguishing some causes of excessive hair loss (see Chapter 13).

Scrape/smear preparations are also used as a diagnostic aid by some dermatologists for the cyto-diagnosis of suspected viral blisters and pemphigus, using a 'Tzanck preparation', which enables material to be examined directly in the clinic.

## Skin biopsy

Skin biopsy is a very important technique in the diagnosis of many skin disorders. In some, it is critical to have confirmation of a clinical diagnosis before embarking on treatment. Good examples of this are skin cancers, bullous disorders, and infections such as tuberculosis and leprosy. In others it is necessary to take a biopsy because clinical information alone has not provided all the answers.

There are two methods commonly used to obtain a skin sample for laboratory examination:

1 Incisional/excisional biopsy
2 Punch biopsy

Specimens obtained by either technique may be sent for conventional histopathology—normally fixed immediately in formol–saline—and/or other specialized examinations, e.g. for DNA phe-notyping of specific cells or for viral DNA. For immunopathology the skin is usually snap frozen. For electron microscopy, skin is best fixed in glutaraldehyde.

Always check the details with the laboratory before you start.

### Incisional/excisional biopsy

This provides good-sized samples (which can be divided for different purposes if required) and can be used to remove quite large lesions (see Figures 2.2 and 2.3).

1 **Administer local anaesthetic:** 1–2% lidocaine is usual; addition of 1:10000 adrenaline (epinephrine) helps reduce bleeding, but never use on fingers and toes
2 **For incisional (diagnostic) biopsy:** make two cuts, forming an ellipse; ensure that the specimen is taken across the edge of the lesion, retaining a margin of normal perilesional skin (Figure 2.2a)
3 **For complete excision:** widen the ellipse around the whole lesion (Figure 2.2b); ensure that the excision edge is cut vertically and *does not* slant in towards the tumour, which can result in inadequate deeper excision (Figure 2.4)
4 **Repair the defect:** edges left by either incisional or excisional biopsy are brought neatly together with sutures; the choice of suture material is not critical, but for the best cosmetic result use the finest possible, preferably a synthetic monofilament suture (e.g. Prolene)

Figure 2.3 Equipment needed for an incisional/excisional biopsy: sterile towel; gauze squares; cotton-wool balls; galley pot containing antiseptic; needle; cartridge of lidocaine and dental syringe; scalpel; skin hook; scissors; small artery forceps; needle holder and suture; fine-toothed forceps; needle and syringe (alternative to dental syringe).

Figure 2.4 Excisional biopsy: the correct (✓) and incorrect (✗) excision edge.

**Note:** if there will be significant tension on the suture line, consider asking a trained plastic or dermatological surgeon for advice.

## Punch biopsy

This is much quicker, but produces small samples (usually 4 or 6 mm in diameter) and is appro-priate only for diagnostic biopsies or removing tiny lesions (Figure 2.5a–c):

1 Administer local anaesthesia (see above)
2 Push the punch biopsy blade into the lesion using a circular motion
3 Lift out the small plug, and separate with scissors or a scalpel blade
4 Achieve haemostasis with silver nitrate, cautery or a small suture

## Patch tests

If a contact allergic dermatitis is suspected, a patch test is performed. In this process possible allergens are usually diluted in suitable vehicles. The test materials are placed in small discs in contact with the skin (usually on the back) for 48 h (Figure 2.6a). A positive reaction (at 48 h, or occa-sionally later) confirms a delayed hypersensitivity (type IV) reaction to the offending substance (Figure 2.6b).

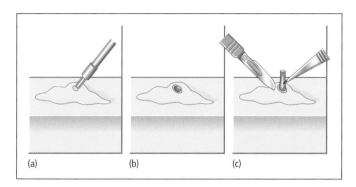

(a)          (b)          (c)

Figure 2.5 The technique for a punch biopsy.

(a)

(b)

Figure 2.6 Patch testing: (a) metal cups containing allergens; (b) positive patch test reactions.

This technique can be extended to include testing for photoallergy.

## Conclusion

You are now ready to start examining and talking to patients with skin disease. Attend some dermatology clinics and put these principles into practice. When seeing patients, try to retain a mental picture of their skin lesions. Ask the dermatologist in charge what the diagnosis is in each instance, and make sure that you read a little about each entity when the clinic is over.

The remaining chapters of this book are designed to help you to make specific diagnoses, to provide your patients with information about their problems and to assist you in choosing appropriate treatment.

# 3

# Bacterial and viral infections

*A mighty creature is the germ*
*Though smaller than the pachyderm*
*His customary dwelling place*
*Is deep within the human race*
*His childish pride he often pleases*
*By giving people strange diseases*
*Do you, my poppet, feel infirm?*
*You probably contain a germ*
                    *Ogden Nash,* The Germ

## Bacterial infections

### Streptococcal infection

#### Cellulitis

Cellulitis is a bacterial infection of subcutaneous tissues that, in immunologically normal individuals, is usually caused by *Streptococcus pyogenes*. 'Erysipelas' is a term applied to superficial streptococcal cellulitis that has a well-demarcated edge. Occasionally, other bacteria are implicated in cellulitis—*Haemophilus influenzae* is an important cause of facial cellulitis in children, often in association with ipsilateral otitis media. In immunocompromised individuals, a variety of bacteria may be responsible for cellulitis.

*Lecture Notes: Dermatology,* 10th edition. © RAC Graham-Brown and DA Burns. Published 2011 by Blackwell Publishing Ltd.

Cellulitis frequently occurs on the legs, but other parts of the body may be affected—the face is a common site for erysipelas. The organisms may gain entry into the skin via minor abrasions, or fissures between the toes associated with tinea pedis, and leg ulcers provide a portal of entry in many cases. A frequent predisposing factor is oedema of the legs, and cellulitis is a common condition in elderly people, who often have leg oedema of cardiac, venous or lymphatic origin.

The affected area becomes red, hot and swollen (Figure 3.1), and blister formation and areas of skin necrosis may occur. The patient is pyrexial and feels unwell. Rigors may occur and, in elderly people, a toxic confusional state.

In presumed streptococcal cellulitis penicillin is the treatment of choice, initially given as benzylpenicillin intravenously. If the leg is affected, bed rest is an important aspect of treatment. Where there is extensive tissue necrosis, surgical debridement may be necessary.

A particularly severe, deep form of cellulitis, involving fascia and muscles, is known as 'necrotizing fasciitis'. This disorder achieved notoriety a few years ago when it attracted the attention of the UK media and was described as being caused by a 'flesh-eating virus'. It is associated with extensive tissue necrosis and severe toxaemia, and is rapidly fatal unless urgent treatment, including excision of the affected area, is undertaken.

Figure 3.1 Cellulitis.

Some patients have recurrent episodes of cellulitis, each episode damaging lymphatics and leading to further oedema. These cases should be treated with prophylactic oral phenoxymethylpenicillin (penicillin V) or erythromycin, to prevent further episodes.

## Staphylococcal infection

### Folliculitis

Infection of the superficial part of a hair follicle with *Staphylococcus aureus* produces a small pustule on an erythematous base, centred on the follicle.

Mild folliculitis can be treated with a topical antibacterial agent, but if it is extensive a systemic antibiotic may be required.

### Furunculosis ('boils')

A boil (furuncle) is the result of deep infection of a hair follicle by *S. aureus*. A painful abscess devel-ops at the site of infection, and over a period of a few days becomes fluctuant and 'points' as a central pustule. Once the necrotic central core has been discharged, the lesion gradually resolves. In some patients boils are a recurrent problem, but this is rarely associated with a significant underlying disorder. Such individuals may be nasal or perineal carriers of staphylococci, and organisms are transferred on the digits to various parts of the body.

Patients suffering from recurrent boils should have swabs taken from the nose for culture, and if found to be carrying staphylococci should be treated with a topical antibacterial such as mupirocin, applied to the nostrils. They may also be helped by an antibacterial bath additive, e.g. 2% triclosan, and a prolonged course of flucloxacillin.

### Carbuncle

A carbuncle is a deep infection of a group of adjacent hair follicles with *S. aureus*. A frequent site for a carbuncle is the nape of the neck. Initially, the lesion is a dome-shaped area of tender erythema, but after a few days suppuration begins, and pus is discharged from multiple follicular orifices. Carbuncles are usually encountered in middle-aged and elderly men, and are associated with diabetes and debility. They are uncommon nowadays. Flucloxacillin should be given for treatment.

### Impetigo

This is a contagious superficial infection that occurs in two clinical forms: non-bullous and bullous. Non-bullous impetigo is caused by *S. aureus*, streptococci or both organisms together. The streptococcal form predominates in warm, humid climates, e.g. the southern USA. Bullous impetigo is caused by *S. aureus*. Lesions may occur anywhere on the body. In the non-bullous form the initial lesion is a small pustule that ruptures to leave an extending area of exudation and crusting (Figure 3.2). The crusts eventually separate to leave areas of erythema, which fade without scarring. In the bullous form, large superficial blisters develop. When these rupture there is exudation and crusting, and the stratum corneum peels back at the edges of the lesions.

Streptococcal impetigo may be associated with poststreptococcal acute glomerulonephritis.

Figure 3.2 Impetigo.

Impetigo may occur as a secondary phenomenon in atopic eczema, scabies and head louse infection.

In localized infection, treatment with a topical antibiotic such as mupirocin will suffice, but in more extensive infection treatment with a systemic antibiotic such as flucloxacillin or erythromycin is indicated.

## Staphylococcal scalded skin syndrome

This uncommon condition occurs as a result of infection with certain staphylococcal phage types that produce a toxin, which splits the epidermis at the level of the granular layer. The superficial epidermis peels off in sheets, producing an appearance resembling scalded skin. Infants and young children are usually affected. It responds to parenteral therapy with flucloxacillin.

## Erythrasma

Caused by a Gram-positive organism, *Corynebacterium minutissimum*, erythrasma occurs in intertriginous areas—axillae, groins and submammary regions. However, the most common site colonized by this organism is the toe-web spaces, where it produces a macerated scaling appearance identical to that caused by fungal infection. In other sites it produces marginated brown areas with a fine, branny, surface scale (Figure 3.3). It is usually asymptomatic. *Corynebacterium minutissimum* produces a porphyrin that fluoresces a striking coral-pink under Wood's light.

Figure 3.3 Erythrasma.

Erythrasma may be treated with topical imidazoles (e.g. clotrimazole, miconazole), topical fusidic acid or a 2-week course of oral erythromycin.

## Mycobacterial infection

### Cutaneous tuberculosis

Cutaneous tuberculosis (TB) is now uncommon in Europe and the USA, but may be encountered in immigrants from other parts of the world where TB remains problematic.

### Scrofuloderma

Scrofuloderma results from involvement of the skin overlying a tuberculous focus, usually a lymph node, most commonly in the neck. The clinical appearance is of multiple fistulae and dense scar tissue.

### Lupus vulgaris

The majority of lesions of lupus vulgaris occur on the head and neck. The typical appearance is of a reddish-brown, nodular plaque (Figure 3.4). When pressed with a glass slide (diascopy), the brown nodules, which are referred to as 'apple jelly' nodules, are more easily seen. The natural course is gradual peripheral extension, and in many cases this is extremely slow, over a period of years. Lupus vulgaris is a destructive process, and the cartilage of the nose and ears may be severely damaged.

Histology shows tubercles composed of epithelioid cells and Langhans' giant cells, usually without central caseation. Tubercle bacilli are sparse. The tuberculin test is strongly positive. The patient should be investigated for an underlying focus of TB in other organs, but this is found only in a small proportion of cases.

Treatment should be with standard antituberculous chemotherapy.

There is a risk of the development of squamous cell carcinoma in the scar tissue of longstanding lupus vulgaris.

### Warty tuberculosis

This occurs as a result of direct inoculation of tubercle bacilli into the skin of someone previously infected, who has a high degree of immunity. It may develop on the buttocks and thighs as a result of sitting on ground contaminated by infected sputum. The clinical appearance is of a warty plaque. It responds to standard antituberculous chemotherapy.

### Tuberculides

This term is applied to skin lesions that occur in response to TB elsewhere in the body. They are probably the result of haematogenous dissemination of bacilli in individuals with a moderate or high degree of immunity.

Included in this group are erythema induratum (Bazin's disease), papulonecrotic tuberculide and lichen scrofulosorum.

Figure 3.4 Lupus vulgaris on the chin.

**Figure 3.5** Fish tank granuloma showing sporotrichoid spread.

## Atypical mycobacteria

The most common of the skin lesions produced by atypical mycobacteria is 'swimming pool' or 'fish tank' granuloma. This is usually a solitary granulomatous nodule, caused by inoculation of *Mycobacterium marinum* into the skin via an abrasion sustained while swimming, or in tropical fish fanciers while cleaning out the aquarium—often after the demise of the fish contained therein. Occasionally, in addition to the initial lesion, there are several secondary lesions in a linear distribution along the lines of lymphatics (sporotrichoid spread—because it resembles sporotrichosis) (Figure 3.5). Most cases respond to treatment with minocycline or doxycycline.

## Leprosy (Hansen's disease)

The Norwegian Armauer Hansen discovered the leprosy bacillus, *Mycobacterium leprae*, in 1873, and, if the possibility of leprosy enters into the discussion of differential diagnosis in the clinic, the eponymous title of this condition should always be used, because the fear of leprosy is so ingrained, even in countries where it is not endemic.

Leprosy has a wide distribution throughout the world, with most cases occurring in the tropics and subtropics, but population movements mean that the disease may be encountered anywhere.

Leprosy is a disease of peripheral nerves, but it also affects the skin, and sometimes other tissues such as the eyes, the mucosa of the upper respiratory tract, the bones and the testes. Although it is infectious, the degree of infectivity is low. The incubation period is lengthy, probably several years, and it is likely that most patients acquire the infection in childhood. A low incidence of conjugal leprosy (leprosy acquired from an infected spouse) suggests that adults are relatively non-susceptible. The disease is acquired as a result of close physical contact with an infected person, the risk being much greater for contacts of lepromatous cases—the nasal discharges of these individuals are the main source of infection in the community.

The clinical pattern of disease is determined by the host's cell-mediated immune response to the organism. When this is well developed tuberculoid leprosy occurs, in which skin and peripheral nerves are affected. Skin lesions are single, or few in number, and are well defined. They are macules or plaques that are hypopigmented in dark skin. The lesions are anaesthetic, sweating is absent and hairs are reduced in number. Thickened branches of cutaneous sensory nerves may be palpable in the region of these lesions, and large peripheral nerves may also be palpable. The lepromin test is strongly positive. Histology shows well-defined tuberculoid granulomas, and bacilli are not seen. The Wade–Fite stain is used to demonstrate leprosy bacilli.

When the cell-mediated immune response is poor, the bacilli multiply unchecked and the patient develops lepromatous leprosy. The bacilli spread to involve not only the skin, but also the mucosa of the respiratory tract, the eyes, testes and bones. Skin lesions are multiple and nodular. The lepromin test is negative. Histology shows a diffuse granuloma throughout the dermis, and bacilli are present in large numbers.

In between these two extreme, 'polar' forms of leprosy is a spectrum of disease referred to as borderline leprosy, the clinical and histological features of which reflect different degrees of cell-mediated response to the bacilli. There is no absolute diagnostic test for leprosy—the diagnosis is based on clinical and histological features.

Cases at the tuberculoid end of the leprosy spectrum (paucibacillary) are treated with a combination of monthly rifampicin and daily dapsone for 6 months, and those at the lepromatous end (multibacillary) with monthly doses of rifampicin and clofazimine, and daily dapsone and clofazimine for 24 months. The treatment of leprosy may be complicated by immunologically mediated 'reactional states', and should be supervised by someone experienced in leprosy management.

---

**The leprosy spectrum**

**Tuberculoid**
- One or two skin lesions only
- Good cell-mediated immune response
- Positive lepromin test
- Few bacilli

**Borderline**
- Scattered skin lesions
- Intermediate cell-mediated immune response
- Some organisms

**Lepromatous**
- Extensive skin lesions and involvement of other organs
- Poor cell-mediated immune response
- Negative lepromin test
- Numerous organisms

---

# Viral infections

## Warts

'Mr Lely, I desire you would use all your skill to paint my picture truly like me, and not flatter me at all; but remark all these roughnesses, pimples, warts, and everything as you see me, otherwise I will never pay a farthing for it.'

Oliver Cromwell to the artist Sir Peter Lely—origin of 'warts and all'

Warts are benign epidermal neoplasms caused by viruses of the human papillomavirus (HPV) group. There are a number of different strains of HPV that produce different clinical types of warts. Warts are also known as 'verrucae', although the term 'verruca' in popular usage is usually reserved for the plantar wart.

## Common warts

These are raised, cauliflower-like lesions that occur most frequently on the hands (Figure 3.6). They are extremely common in childhood and early adult life. They may be scattered, grouped or periungual in distribution. Common warts in children usually resolve spontaneously.

Common warts are usually treated with wart paints or cryotherapy. Preparations containing salicylic acid are often quite effective, and a wart paint should certainly be used for at least 3 months before considering alternative treatment.

Cryotherapy with liquid nitrogen can be used on warts that do not respond to wart paints. A simple applicator of cotton wool wrapped around the end of an orange stick may be used. This is dipped in the liquid nitrogen and then applied to the wart until it and a narrow rim of surrounding skin are frozen. Alternatively, a liquid nitrogen cryospray may be used. This is a painful procedure, and should not be inflicted on children—however, most tiny tots will, sensibly, retreat under the desk protesting loudly at first sight of the nitrogen evaporating in its container. Multiple warts usually require more than one application, and the optimum interval between treatments is 2–3 weeks.

## Plantar warts

Plantar warts may be solitary, scattered over the sole of the foot, or grouped together producing so-called 'mosaic' warts (Figure 3.7). The typical appearance is of a small area of thickened skin which, when pared away, reveals numerous small black dots produced by thrombosed capillaries. Plantar warts are frequently painful. They must be distinguished from calluses and corns, which develop in areas of friction over bony prominences. Calluses are patches of uniformly thick-

Figure 3.6 Viral warts.

Figure 3.7 Mosaic plantar warts.

ened skin, and corns have a painful central plug of keratin that does not contain capillaries.

Treatment is with wart paints or cryotherapy, after paring down overlying keratin.

## Plane warts

These are tiny, flat-topped, flesh-coloured warts which usually occur on the dorsa of the hands and the face (Figure 3.8). They often occur in lines due to inoculation of the virus into scratches and abrasions. Plane warts are extremely difficult to treat effectively, and attempts at treatment may do more harm than good. They will resolve spontaneously eventually, and are best left alone.

## Genital warts (condylomata acuminata)

In recent years the importance of certain types of genital wart viruses in the aetiology of penile and cervical cancer has been recognized, and this has modified attitudes to what was previously considered a minor sexually transmitted inconvenience. It is now more appropriate that patients with genital warts are seen and treated in a department of genitourinary medicine, so that coexisting sexually transmitted infection may be detected and treated, and sexual contacts traced and examined.

Figure 3.8 Plane warts.

Figure 3.9 Molluscum contagiosum.

## Molluscum contagiosum

The lesions of molluscum contagiosum are caused by a poxvirus. They are typically pearly, pink papules with a central umbilication filled with a keratin plug (Figure 3.9). The lesions may occur anywhere on the body, but are most common on the head and neck area and the trunk. They are frequently grouped, and may be surrounded by a mild eczematous reaction. They may be very extensive in children with atopic eczema.

These lesions resolve spontaneously, and in infants and small children are best left alone to do so. However, if parents of small children are anxious they can be advised to squeeze each lesion between the thumbnails to express the central plug—this will often speed their resolution. In older children and adults molluscum contagiosum can be treated by cryotherapy.

## Orf

Orf is caused by a parapoxvirus. It is a disease of sheep that can be transmitted to humans. Those usually affected are people who bottle-feed lambs, and butchers and abattoir workers who handle the carcasses of sheep. The typical clinical picture is of a solitary, inflammatory papule that rapidly develops into a nodule of granulation tissue—usually on a finger, but occasionally on the face. The diagnosis can be confirmed by electron microscopy of smears from the granulation tissue. Orf lesions resolve spontaneously in 6–8 weeks, but the disease may act as a trigger for erythema multiforme.

## Hand, foot and mouth disease

This is not related to foot and mouth disease of sheep and cattle, but is a harmless disease caused by Coxsackie virus infection, usually type A16. Characteristic small grey vesicles with a halo of

Figure 3.10 Hand, foot and mouth disease: vesicles on the hand.

erythema occur on the hands and feet (Figure 3.10), and the buccal mucosa is studded with erosions resembling aphthous ulcers. The condition resolves within 2 weeks, and no treatment is required.

## Herpes simplex

Herpes simplex is caused by herpesvirus hominis (herpes simplex virus, HSV). There are two antigenic types: type 1 is classically associated with the common 'cold sore' on the lips and face, and type 2 with genital herpes. However, neither has rigid territorial demarcation, and lesions anywhere may be caused by either antigenic type.

### Primary herpes simplex

Initial contact with type 1 HSV usually occurs in early childhood, e.g. adults with cold sores kissing children, and any lesions that develop are often so mild that they are not noticed. Occasionally, however, a severe primary herpetic gingivostomatitis occurs, with painful erosions on the buccal mucosa and lips. Primary cutaneous herpes simplex may also occur, and in atopic eczema this can be very extensive and may be life threatening (see below). Genital herpes may result from sexual transmission of type 2 HSV or orogenital transmission of type 1 HSV.

Physical contact during sport provides another means of HSV transmission—in rugby, herpes simplex thus acquired is known as 'scrumpox', and in wrestling as 'herpes gladiatorum'.

Following a primary infection the virus settles in sensory ganglia, and may be triggered to produce recurrent lesions by a variety of stimuli. In immunodeficient individuals, e.g. those who are immunosuppressed after organ transplantation, or in association with human immunodeficiency virus (HIV) infection, herpes simplex infection may be clinically atypical and run a prolonged course.

### Recurrent herpes simplex

Recurrent cold sores on the lips (herpes labialis) are common. Itching and discomfort in the affected area precede, by a few hours, the eruption of a group of small vesicles. The vesicle contents subsequently become cloudy, and then crusting occurs, before resolution in about 10 days. The trigger for these episodes is often fever, but exposure to strong sunlight and menstruation are also recognized precipitants. Occasionally, as a result of inoculation of the virus into a finger, painful episodes of 'herpetic whitlow' occur. The frequency of episodes of herpes simplex usually declines gradually with advancing age.

Labial herpes simplex is usually a minor cosmetic inconvenience, and does not require treatment. However, if episodes are frequent and troublesome, topical aciclovir may be of benefit. This blocks viral replication—it is not viricidal and is not curative.

Figure 3.11 Eczema herpeticum.

## Herpes simplex and erythema multiforme

Recurrent herpes simplex can trigger erythema multiforme. Prophylactic oral aciclovir may be of considerable benefit in the management of severe cases.

## Eczema herpeticum (Kaposi's varicelliform eruption)

This is a widespread herpes simplex infection that occurs in atopic eczema. The head and neck are frequently affected (Figure 3.11), but lesions may spread rapidly to involve extensive areas of skin. Lymphadenopathy and constitutional upset may occur. If the disease is limited in distribution and the patient is seen early in its course, oral aciclovir therapy is appropriate. However, if the lesions are extensive, and the patient is unwell, they should be admitted to hospital and treated with intravenous aciclovir. If the patient is using topical steroid therapy to treat the eczema, this should be stopped until the herpes has resolved. Eczema herpeticum may recur, but in many cases subsequent episodes tend to be less severe.

## Herpes zoster (shingles)

Chickenpox and herpes zoster are both caused by the varicella-zoster virus. 'Shingles' is a distortion of the Latin *cingulum*, meaning a girdle.

Following an attack of chickenpox the virus remains dormant in dorsal root ganglia until some stimulus reactivates it and causes shingles.

Middle aged and elderly people are most often affected, but it occasionally occurs in childhood. It is also more frequent in immunosuppressed individuals.

Shingles usually affects a single dermatome, most commonly on the thorax or abdomen. The eruption may be preceded by pain in the region of the dermatome, and this occasionally leads to an incorrect diagnosis of internal pathology. The lesions consist of a unilateral band of grouped vesicles on an erythematous base (Figure 3.12). The contents of the vesicles are initially clear, but subsequently become cloudy. There may be scattered outlying vesicles on the rest of the body, and these tend to be more numerous in elderly people. However, numerous outlying vesicles (disseminated zoster) are also seen in immunosuppressed individuals, and their presence should prompt further investigation of the patient. After a few days the vesicles dry up and form crusts, and in most cases the eruption resolves within 2 weeks. In elderly people, shingles can produce quite severe erosive changes that take considerably longer to heal. Even in milder cases there is usually some residual scarring.

The most troublesome aspect of shingles is the persistence of pain after the lesions have healed (postherpetic neuralgia). This may be severe, and is particularly distressing for elderly people.

## Sacral zoster

Involvement of the sacral segments may cause acute retention of urine in association with the rash.

Figure 3.12 Herpes zoster.

## Trigeminal zoster

Herpes zoster may affect any of the divisions of the trigeminal nerve, but the ophthalmic division is the most frequently involved (Figure 3.13). Ocular problems such as conjunctivitis, keratitis and/or iridocyclitis may occur if the nasociliary branch of the ophthalmic division is affected (indicated by vesicles on the side of the nose [Hutchinson's sign]), and patients with ophthalmic zoster should be examined by an ophthalmologist.

Involvement of the maxillary division of the trigeminal nerve produces vesicles on the cheek, and unilateral vesicles on the palate.

## Motor zoster

Occasionally, in addition to skin lesions in a sensory dermatome, motor fibres are affected, leading to muscle weakness.

## Treatment of herpes zoster

Many cases do not require any treatment. However, in severe cases, and in all cases of ophthalmic zoster, oral aciclovir, valaciclovir or famciclovir should be given. In disseminated zoster in immunosuppressed individuals, intravenous aciclovir can be life saving.

Pain relief is often difficult to achieve in postherpetic neuralgia, and patients with severe discomfort should be referred to a pain relief specialist.

Figure 3.13 Ophthalmic zoster.

# 4

# Fungal infections

The fungi that may cause human disease include the dermatophytes (Greek, meaning 'skin plants') and the yeast-like fungus *Candida albicans*, which are responsible for superficial fungal infections confined to the skin, hair and nails, and mucous membranes. Other fungi can invade living tissue to cause deep infections, which may remain localized (mycetoma) or cause systemic disease (e.g. histoplasmosis).

The dermatophytes are a group of fungi that are responsible for so-called 'ringworm' infections. The vegetative phase of dermatophyte fungi consists of septate hyphae which form a branching network (mycelium). *Candida albicans* is an organism composed of round or oval cells which divide by budding. Apart from its yeast form it may produce pseudohyphae consisting of numerous cells in a linear arrangement or, in certain circumstances, true septate hyphae.

## Dermatophyte infections

It is very easy to become totally confused by the terminology employed in fungal infection, and end up not knowing your tinea cruris from your *Trichophyton rubrum*. Hence, a novice is best advised to stick to simple terminology. The term 'ringworm', followed by 'of the feet, of the groin, of the scalp', etc., is a simple way of indicating the location of the infection. If you feel in more classical mood you may use 'tinea' (Latin, meaning 'a gnawing worm') followed by 'pedis, cruris, capitis', etc.

*Lecture Notes: Dermatology*, 10th edition. © RAC Graham-Brown and DA Burns. Published 2011 by Blackwell Publishing Ltd.

The dermatophyte fungi are named according to their genus (*Microsporum*, *Trichophyton* and *Epidermophyton*) and their species (e.g. *M. canis*, *T. rubrum*), and they can be distinguished from each other in culture. An experienced dermatologist may be able to suggest that a certain fungus is responsible for a particular case of ringworm, but the only way to establish its identity precisely is by culture.

Some fungi are confined to humans (anthropophilic); others principally affect animals (zoophilic) but occasionally infect humans. When animal fungi cause human skin lesions their presence often provokes a severe inflammatory reaction (e.g. cattle ringworm). Dermatophytes grow only in keratin—the stratum corneum of the skin, hair and nails. Infection is usually acquired by contact with keratin debris carrying fungal hyphae, e.g. the woman who developed ringworm on the buttocks as a result of her husband's habit of cutting his toenails with his feet resting on the lavatory seat.

### Tinea pedis (athlete's foot)

This is the most common of the dermatophyte infections, and usually presents as scaling, itchy areas in the toe webs, particularly between the third and fourth and fourth and fifth toes, or on the soles (Figure 4.1). It is usually acquired from contact with infected keratin debris on the floors of swimming pools and showers. Sometimes there is extensive involvement of the soles and sides of the feet (so-called moccasin tinea pedis, because of its similarity to the shape of that soft leather shoe). The condition may also spread on to the dorsa of the feet.

Figure 4.1 Athlete's foot.

Figure 4.2 Tinea cruris.

Occasionally, athlete's foot follows a pattern of episodic vesiculobullous lesions on the soles, occurring particularly during warm weather. The feet are frequently asymmetrically involved in fungal infection, in contrast with eczema, in which the involvement is usually symmetrical.

## Tinea cruris

This is common in men and rare in women. The clinical picture is characteristic, and should be easy to distinguish from intertrigo, flexural psoriasis and flexural seborrhoeic dermatitis. A scaly, erythematous margin gradually spreads down the medial aspects of the thighs (Figure 4.2), and may extend backwards to involve the perineum and buttocks. The source of the infection is nearly always the patient's feet, so they should be examined for evidence of athlete's foot or fungal nail dystrophy. The fungus is presumably transferred to the groins on fingers that have scratched itchy feet and then scratched groins, or on towels.

## Tinea corporis

Tinea on the body typically has an inflammatory edge with central clearing (Figure 4.3), but it is relatively uncommon. The differential diagnosis includes granuloma annulare and erythema annulare. In the former there is a raised margin, but no scaling. The latter provides more diagnostic difficulty because the inflammatory margin is scaly. If fungal infection is suspected, scrapings should be examined microscopically for hyphae. In adults, the source of the fungus is usually the feet, whereas in children it has usually spread from the scalp.

## Tinea manuum

Ringworm on the hand is usually unilateral. On the palm the appearance is of mild scaling erythema, whereas on the dorsum there is more obvious inflammatory change, with a well-defined edge (Figure 4.4). The source of the fungus is almost invariably the patient's feet.

Figure 4.3 Tinea corporis.

Figure 4.4 Tinea on the dorsum of the hand. Note involvement of middle finger nail.

## Tinea unguium

Toenail fungal dystrophy is very common in adults, and is invariably associated with athlete's foot. The involvement usually starts laterally as yellowish streaks in the nail plate (Figure 4.5), but gradually the whole nail becomes thickened, discoloured and friable. *T. rubrum* is usually the cause. The great toenails are often the first to be affected, and pressure from footwear on the thickened nails may produce considerable discomfort.

A less common pattern is white superficial onychomycosis, in which the dorsal part of the nail plate shows white patches, and *T. mentagrophytes* is usually responsible for this.

Rapid proximal invasion of the nail plate, producing white discoloration, is a pattern seen in AIDS patients.

Fingernails are less commonly affected. The changes in the nail plate are similar to those seen in toenails (Figure 4.6).

## Tinea capitis

Tinea capitis is principally a disease of childhood, and is rare in adults. This is thought to be related to a change in the fatty acid constituents of sebum around the time of puberty. Postpubertal sebum contains fungistatic fatty acids. The principal fungi responsible for scalp ringworm vary in different parts of the world. In the UK, until recent years, most cases of scalp ringworm were the result of *M. canis* infection, usually acquired from cats, but immigration has led to the appearance of other scalp ringworm organisms. In the USA the usual causative organism is *Trichophyton tonsurans*, and in the Indian subcontinent the most common cause is *T. violaceum*.

One or more patches of partial hair loss develop on an otherwise normal scalp (Figure 4.7). The affected scalp is scaly, and the hair is usually broken off just above the surface, producing irregular stubble. In some cases there is little obvious

Figure 4.5 Tinea of the toenails.

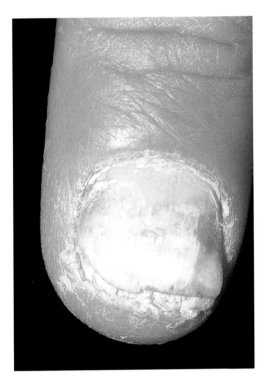

Figure 4.6 Tinea of a fingernail.

inflammation, but in others this is prominent and there is pustule formation.

Occasionally the area of scalp involved is more extensive, producing an appearance suggestive of seborrhoeic dermatitis. *Microsporum canis* fluoresces yellow–green under long-wavelength ultraviolet light (Wood's light)—see Chapter 2.

## Kerion

Kerion (Greek, meaning 'honeycomb') is a term applied to severe inflammatory scalp ringworm, usually provoked by the fungus of cattle ringworm, but occasionally by other fungi. It resembles a bacterial infection, with pustules and abscesses (Figure 4.8), and affected children are often given repeated courses of antibiotics on this assumption. They may also be subjected to surgical incision of the areas.

## Cattle ringworm

In rural areas, young farm workers often have cattle ringworm—older farmers have usually had the disease, and develop immunity against reinfection. The face and forearms are the areas most frequently affected. There is a marked inflammatory reaction to the fungus, producing an appearance resembling a bacterial infection (Figure 4.9).

Children who visit farms may pick up the fungus from gates and fences where cattle have left keratin debris containing the organism, and subsequently develop a kerion.

## Tinea incognito

This term is applied to a fungal infection, the appearance of which has been altered by inappropriate treatment with topical steroid preparations. Topical steroids suppress the inflammatory response to the fungus, and the typical scaly erythematous margin usually disappears, leaving an ill-defined area of patchy scaling erythema studded with pustules.

Figure 4.7 Scalp ringworm.

Figure 4.8 Kerion.

## 'Ide' reactions

Patients suffering from the florid vesicular type of athlete's foot may develop an acute vesiculobullous eruption on the hands known as an 'ide' reaction. The appearance is indistinguishable from the acute eczematous response known as pompholyx (see Chapter 7). The lesions on the hands do not contain fungus. The reaction appears to have an immunological basis, but the exact pathomechanism is unknown. Occasionally, a more generalized maculopapular ide reaction accompanies a fungal infection.

## Diagnosis

Skin scrapings, nail clippings and plucked hair can be examined as described in Chapter 2. A little experience is necessary to distinguish fungal mycelium (Figure 4.10) from cell walls and intercellular lipid, or filamentous debris. Fungal mycelium has the appearance of long rows of railway wagons which branch periodically. Material may also be sent to the mycology laboratory for culture.

## Treatment

There are a number of topical antifungal agents available for the treatment of dermatophyte infections, including miconazole, clotrimazole, econazole, sulconazole and terbinafine. These can be used when small areas of skin are affected, but if a fungal infection is extensive it is preferable to employ an oral agent such as griseofulvin, terbinafine or itraconazole—in adults, griseofulvin

500 mg daily for 2–4 weeks, terbinafine 250 mg daily for 2–4 weeks or itraconazole 100 mg daily for 15–30 days.

Topical agents alone are not effective in scalp ringworm, which should be treated with an oral agent—griseofulvin or terbinafine for 4–6 weeks. Although it is not licensed for use in children in the UK, many dermatologists prefer to use terbinafine for the treatment of scalp ringworm. Dosages of oral agents are calculated according to the child's weight. To reduce the risk of transmission of scalp ringworm organisms from child to child, a topical agent such as an antifungal shampoo (selenium sulfide, ketoconazole) should be used in combination with oral therapy, to kill organisms on the surface of the scalp.

The treatment of choice for nail infections is oral terbinafine—250 mg daily for 6 weeks in fingernail infections and for 3 months in toenail infections. An alternative is itraconazole pulse therapy—200 mg twice daily for 7 days; for fingernails, repeat once after a 3-week drug-free interval; for toenails, repeat twice with a 3-week drug-free interval between each course. Various combination therapies, e.g. oral terbinafine plus topical amorolfine nail lacquer, have been suggested in attempts to increase cure rates and reduce costs of treatment.

Figure 4.9 Cattle ringworm on the forearm of a farmer.

## Mycetoma (Madura foot)

In certain parts of the world, e.g. the Indian subcontinent, trauma to the feet may result in the inoculation of certain soil fungi, which produce a deep-seated chronic infection with abscesses and draining sinuses. The causative organisms are often unresponsive to systemic antifungal agents.

Figure 4.10 Fungal mycelium.

# Candida infection

Candidiasis (moniliasis, 'thrush') is a term applied to infections of the skin and mucous membranes by yeast-like fungi of the genus *Candida*. The most common, *Candida albicans*, is a normal commensal of the human digestive tract, where it exists in balance with the bacterial flora. In its commensal role, *Candida* sp. is present as budding yeasts. In a pathogenic role, budding and mycelial forms are usually present. It becomes pathogenic only when situations favourable to its multiplication arise. These include topical and systemic steroid therapy, immunosuppression of any aetiology (e.g. lymphoma, AIDS), broad-spectrum antibiotic therapy, diabetes mellitus, and the apposition of areas of skin to produce a warm, moist environment.

The diagnosis of candidiasis can be confirmed by culture of swabs taken from the affected areas.

## Buccal mucosal candidiasis

White, curd-like plaques adhere to the buccal mucosa. If these are scraped off, the underlying epithelium is inflamed and friable. It may be treated with nystatin oral suspension, amphotericin lozenges, miconazole oral gel or itraconazole liquid.

## Angular cheilitis (perléche)

Angular cheilitis is an inflammatory process occurring at the corners of the mouth (Figure 4.11). The main factors involved in its causation, either alone or in combination, include infection with *Candida* sp. or staphylococci, and the development of prominent creases at the angles of the mouth, either as a normal consequence of age or in edentulous individuals who do not wear dentures or have ill-fitting dentures. Saliva is drawn into the creases by capillary action, and salivary enzymes macerate the skin, producing sore, moist areas.

In denture wearers, modification of the dentures may help. Treatment with an imidazole/hydrocortisone combination, e.g. miconazole/hydrocortisone, is usually of benefit.

## Chronic paronychia

This is a chronic inflammatory process affecting the proximal nail fold and nail matrix. It occurs predominantly in those whose hands are repeatedly immersed in water—housewives, bar staff, florists, fishmongers. A sharp decline in the incidence of this disorder in recent years is probably related to more widespread use of mechanical dishwashers, rather than the human variety, and hand protection with washing-up gloves.

The clinical appearance is of thickening and erythema of the proximal nail fold ('bolstering'), and loss of the cuticle (Figure 4.12). There is often an associated nail dystrophy. *Candida albicans* plays a pathogenic role, but bacteria may also be involved. The absence of the cuticle allows access of irritant substances, such as detergents, to the area beneath the proximal nail fold, and this probably contributes to the inflammatory process.

Figure 4.11 Angular cheilitis.

This condition is quite distinct from acute bacterial paronychia, in which there is a short history, severe discomfort and ample production of green pus. Pressure on the swollen nail fold in chronic paronychia may produce a tiny bead of creamy pus from under the nail fold, but that is all.

Treatment consists of advice to keep the hands as dry as possible by wearing cotton-lined rubber or PVC gloves when working, and topical anti-candida therapy, for example with an imidazole.

## Balanoposthitis/vulvovaginitis

Small white patches or eroded areas are present on the foreskin and glans of the uncircumcised penis. Predisposing factors are poor penile hygiene and diabetes mellitus. Candida balanoposthitis may be a recurrent problem if a sexual partner has candida vaginitis.

Candida vulvovaginitis presents with a creamy vaginal discharge and itchy erythema of the vulva. Pregnancy, oral contraceptives and diabetes mellitus are predisposing factors. Balanoposthitis and vulvitis should be treated with a topical anti-candida preparation, and there are several products available to treat vaginal candidiasis.

Don't forget to test the urine for sugar in anyone with candida balanoposthitis or vulvovaginitis.

## Intertrigo

'Intertrigo' is a term applied to maceration that occurs where two skin surfaces are in apposition—groins, axillae, submammary regions or beneath an abdominal fat apron. Obesity and poor hygiene are contributory factors. Candida superinfection is often present, and is suggested clinically by the presence of creamy 'satellite' pustules at the margins of the affected areas. The pustules are easily ruptured, leaving a collarette of scale, and

Figure 4.12 Chronic paronychia.

Figure 4.13 Pityriasis versicolor.

this gives a characteristic scalloped edge to the area of intertrigo.

Therapy with a combined topical preparation containing an anti-candida agent, such as miconazole, and hydrocortisone is usually beneficial, but attention to hygiene is also important.

# Pityriasis versicolor

This condition occurs predominantly in young adults, and is caused by yeasts of the genus *Malassezia*, which are normal skin commensals present in pilosebaceous follicles. It is a common disorder in temperate zones and is seen even more frequently in tropical climates. The reason why these yeasts multiply and produce skin lesions in certain individuals is unknown.

On a fair skin, the lesions are light-brown macules with a fine surface scale (Figures 4.13 and 4.14), and they occur predominantly on the trunk and upper arms. They are usually asymptomatic, but are a cosmetic nuisance. On pigmented skin the typical appearance is of patchy hypopigmentation (Figure 4.15). The loss of pigment is thought to be related to production of azelaic acid by the yeasts, which inhibits tyrosinase and thereby interferes with melanin production. The colour variation, depending on the background skin colour, is the reason for the 'versicolor' in the name.

The diagnosis can be confirmed by microscopic examination of skin scrapings in a mixture of 10% potassium hydroxide and Parker Quink ink (Figure 4.16), when characteristic clumps of round spores and short, stubby hyphae can be seen (an appearance that has been called 'spaghetti and meatballs').

A simple treatment is selenium sulfide, in the form of a shampoo (Selsun), left on the skin for a

Figure 4.15 Hypopigmented pityriasis versicolor on a pigmented skin.

Figure 4.14 Close view of pityriasis versicolor showing fine 'branny' scale.

Figure 4.16 Spores and hyphae of *Malassezia* sp. in pityriasis versicolor.

few minutes during bathing. This will usually clear the organism in 2–3 weeks. Topical imidazole antifungal creams and ketoconazole shampoo are also effective against *Malassezia* sp., as is topical terbinafine. Oral itraconazole is an alternative (200 mg daily for 7 days). Griseofulvin and oral terbinafine are ineffective.

Pityriasis versicolor tends to recur, and treatment may have to be repeated. Hypopigmented areas may take a considerable time to repigment, and their persistence should not be taken as evidence of treatment failure.

# 5

# Ectoparasite infections

## Scabies

*There's a squeak of pure delight from a matey little mite,*
*As it tortuously tunnels in the skin,*
*Singing furrow, folly furrow, come and join me in my burrow,*
*And we'll view the epidermis from within*

Guy's Acarus

### Aetiology

Scabies (Latin = the scab, mange, itch) is caused by small, eight-legged mites (*Sarcoptes scabiei*), and is acquired by close physical contact with another individual with the disease—prolonged hand holding is probably the usual means of spread. Any age group may be affected. It is common in children and young adults, and in recent years has become troublesome in elderly people in residential care homes. Transient contact is not sufficient for spread of classic scabies, and anyone encountering ordinary cases of scabies in a healthcare setting should not be afraid of acquiring the disease.

The female scabies mite burrows in the epidermis, and lays eggs in the burrow behind her. The only function of male scabies mites appears to be to fertilize the females, and then they expire. Initially, the host is unaware of the mining activity in the epidermis, but after a period of 4–6 weeks hypersensitivity to the mite or its products develops, and itching begins. The asymptomatic period is obviously very useful to the parasite because it

*Lecture Notes: Dermatology*, 10th edition. © RAC Graham-Brown and DA Burns. Published 2011 by Blackwell Publishing Ltd.

has time to establish itself before the host response develops. Thereafter, life becomes hazardous for the mites because burrows will be excoriated and mites and eggs destroyed. In this way the host keeps the mite population in check, and in most individuals with scabies the average number of adult female mites on the skin is no more than a dozen.

### Clinical features

The patient complains of itching, which is characteristically worse at night. Scabies should be considered in anyone presenting with this history.

There are two principal types of skin lesion in scabies—burrows and the scabies 'rash'. Burrows are found principally on the hands and feet—the sides of the fingers and toes, the web spaces between digits, the wrists and the insteps. In infants, burrows are often present on the palms of the hands and soles of the feet, and may also be present on the trunk and the head and neck. Burrows on the trunk are a common finding in immobile elderly patients, and they may also occur on the head and neck. Each burrow is several millimetres long, usually tortuous, with a vesicle at one end adjacent to the burrowing mite, and often surrounded by mild erythema (Figure 5.1). Burrows also occur on the male genitalia, usually surmounting inflammatory papules, and these papules on the penis and scrotum are pathognomonic of scabies. If scabies is suspected in a male, the genitalia should always be examined.

The 'rash' of scabies is an eruption of tiny inflammatory papules that occur mainly around the axillae and umbilicus, and on the thighs (Figure 5.2). The rash is an allergic reaction to the mites.

3x

Figure 5.1 Typical scabies burrow.

Figure 5.2 The scabies 'rash'.

In addition to these primary skin lesions, there may be secondary changes such as excoriations, eczematization and secondary bacterial infection. In some parts of the world, secondary infection of scabies lesions with nephritogenic streptococci is associated with the development of poststreptococcal glomerulonephritis.

## Diagnosis

Absolute confirmation of the diagnosis can be made only by demonstrating the mites or eggs microscopically. In order to do this, burrows must be found, and this usually requires some expertise. Look carefully, in good light, at the hands and feet. A magnifying glass or dermatoscope may be of considerable help, but myopia is a distinct

natural advantage. Once a burrow, or a suspected burrow, has been identified, it should be gently scraped off the skin with the edge of a scalpel blade—dermatologists sometimes use a blunt scalpel known as a 'banana' scalpel for this task (see Chapter 2). The scrapings should be placed on a microscope slide with a few drops of 10% potassium hydroxide, covered with a coverslip, and examined under the microscope. The presence of mites, eggs or even eggshells confirms the diagnosis (Figure 5.3). Do not attempt to scrape any lesions on the penis—the proximity of a scalpel to this area leads to understandable apprehension, and is in any case rarely rewarded by the demonstration of mites.

Figure 5.3 Scabies mite and eggs in potassium hydroxide preparation.

## Treatment

*Scabies is treated by eating young alligators and washing the skin with urine. (Mexican folk medicine)*

It is important to explain to patients precisely how to use their treatment, and written explanatory treatment sheets are useful. All family members, and close physical contacts of an affected individual, should be treated simultaneously. Topical agents should be applied from the neck to the toes, and patients should be reminded not to wash their hands after applying treatment. In infants, and elderly and immunocompromised patients, in whom burrows can occur on the head and neck, it may be necessary to extend application to these areas. Itching does not resolve immediately after treatment, but will improve gradually over 2–3 weeks as the superficial epidermis, containing the allergenic mites, is shed. A topical antipruritic such as crotamiton 10% with hydrocortisone 0.25% can be used on residual itchy areas. It is not necessary to 'disinfest' clothing and soft furnishings—laundering of underwear and nightclothes is all that is required.

## Available treatments

### Malathion 0.5%

Aqueous preparations are preferred because they do not irritate excoriated or eczematized skin. Wash off after 24 h.

## Permethrin cream 5%

Wash off after 8–12 h.

A single application of malathion or permethrin is often effective, but a second application 7 days later is recommended.

## Benzylbenzoate emulsion

Although superseded by malathion and permethrin in some parts of the world, in many countries benzylbenzoate is still used to treat scabies because it is effective and inexpensive. One regimen involves three applications in a 24-h period. On the evening of day 1 apply the emulsion from the neck to the toes. Allow to dry, then apply a second coat. The following morning apply a third coat, and then wash off the benzylbenzoate on the evening of day 2. Treatment is then complete, and this should be stressed to the patient because repeated use will produce an irritant dermatitis.

Irritancy is its main drawback.

## Treatment of infants

As burrows can occur on the head and neck it may be necessary to extend application of topical therapy to these areas. The treatment of choice is permethrin.

As a result of the availability of non-irritant agents, benzylbenzoate is not recommended for use in infants, but if it is employed it should be diluted to reduce its irritancy.

## Treatment in pregnancy

There is understandable concern about potential toxic effects on the fetus of scabicides when used in pregnancy. However, there is no definitive evidence that any of the currently employed topical scabicides has been responsible for harmful effects in pregnancy after appropriate use. Hence, in the absence of evidence of fetal toxicity, use of malathion or permethrin appears to be safe.

# Crusted (Norwegian) scabies

This is an uncommon type of scabies in which enormous numbers of mites are present in crusted lesions on the skin. It was called Norwegian scabies because it was originally described in Norwegian individuals with leprosy, but the term 'crusted' is now preferred. The mite is exactly the same as that causing ordinary scabies. Mites are present in such huge numbers because of an altered host response to their presence. Crusted scabies may develop when itching is not perceived because of sensory loss from neurological disorders (hence its occurrence in those with leprosy), in individuals who are immunosuppressed, as a result of either disease (e.g. AIDS) or treatment (e.g. systemic steroids, organ transplantation), or when patients are unable to scratch because of severe rheumatoid arthritis or paresis. In these circumstances, when the host does not itch or cannot scratch, burrows are not destroyed and the mite population multiplies unchecked. Crusted scabies also occurs more frequently in individuals with Down's syndrome.

The crusted skin lesions can contain millions of mites and eggs, and these are shed into the environment on flakes of keratin. Anyone coming into contact with a patient with crusted scabies is at risk of acquiring ordinary scabies, and undiagnosed cases may be responsible for outbreaks of scabies in hospitals and residential homes.

## Clinical features

The hands and feet are usually encased in a thick fissured crust, and areas of crusting may be present on other parts of the body, including the head and neck. The nails are often grossly thickened (Figure 5.4). The changes may resemble psoriatic scaling or hyperkeratotic eczema, and this can lead to the diagnosis being missed. Burrows are usually impossible to identify in the crusted areas, but may be found on less severely affected parts of the body. Microscopy of the scales reveals numerous mites and eggs.

## Treatment

The patient should be isolated, and nurses responsible for their care should wear gowns and gloves. All medical staff and carers, and any other individuals who have been in contact with the patient before diagnosis and treatment, should be treated with a topical scabicide.

Crusted scabies is often difficult to cure with topical agents alone, and usually requires several

Figure 5.4 Crusted scabies in a youth with Down's syndrome.

applications of a scabicide. The current recommended treatment for crusted scabies is a combination of ivermectin (given as a single dose of 200 μg/kg body weight, repeated after an interval of 7 days) with a topical scabicide, applied to the whole body, including the head and neck. Ivermectin is not licensed for use in the treatment of scabies in humans, but may be obtained on a named-patient basis from the manufacturer. It has been used for many years as a treatment for onchocerciasis (river blindness) and other types of filariasis, and is employed in veterinary practice to deal with several types of animal parasites.

## Institutional outbreaks of scabies

The huge increase in the number of residential care and nursing homes for elderly people in the UK in recent years has been associated with numerous outbreaks of scabies in these facilities. Although some are related to cases of crusted scabies, others appear to originate from residents who have a large mite population, or from infected carers. Close contact between residents and carers in these homes is common—carers usually hold the hands of residents to provide support when walking, and this facilitates spread of the disease.

All residents, their carers and the carers' families should be treated with a topical scabicide. Residents who have very numerous burrows, or have crusted scabies, will require more intensive treatment and preferably should be isolated until cured. If such individuals are not identified there is a risk that they may only partially respond to treatment and therefore provide a source for a further outbreak. Ivermectin may prove to be of value in dealing with outbreaks of scabies in residential homes and similar communities.

---

# Pediculosis

## Head lice (*Pediculus capitis*)

*Her ladyship said when I went to her house,*
*That she did not esteem me three skips of a louse;*
*I freely forgave what the dear creature said,*
*For ladies will talk of what runs in their head.*
*Theodore Hook*

Head lice are wingless insects that live on the scalp and feed on blood. Adult head lice are 2–4 mm in length. They are acquired by head-to-head contact with another infected individual. It is still a commonly held belief that head lice are associated with poor hygiene, perhaps supported by the findings of surveys in the earlier part of the twentieth century which showed that head louse infection was principally a problem of the lower classes in large industrial conurbations. However, in more recent years, the head louse has climbed the social ladder and taken up rural pursuits, and is now widely distributed in all socioeconomic groups.

The adult female louse lays eggs that she cements to hair shafts (Figure 5.5). The eggs are

**Figure 5.5** Head louse eggs cemented to a hair shaft.

Figure 5.7 The head louse.

Figure 5.6 Head louse eggs and egg cases.

flesh coloured and difficult to see, but once the louse nymph has emerged (after about 10 days) the empty egg case (nit) is more readily visible.

## Clinical features

Itching is the main symptom. Nits tend to be more numerous in the occipital region of the scalp and above the ears (Figure 5.6). Occasionally, flakes of dandruff or keratin casts around hair shafts may be mistaken for nits, but the distinction is obvious if the material is examined microscopically. Adult lice and nymphs will be found without difficulty in heavier infections (Figure 5.7). Impetigo may occur as a result of inoculation of staphylococci into the skin during scratching; the term 'nitwit' is derived from the substandard performance of children who had large head louse populations, secondary skin sepsis and probably also anaemia, and were chronically unwell as a result.

## Treatment

The approach to treatment has changed in recent years, and it is now considered appropriate to employ a strategy that includes both physical and chemical methods. Chemical means of control, employing insecticides, have been widely used throughout the world, because insecticides are easy to use and convenient, and they have proved very effective. However, there is concern about potential adverse effects, particularly from residual insecticides such as lindane (which is no longer used in some parts of the world, including the UK), not only on humans but also on the environment. In addition, there is evidence of widespread resistance of head lice to malathion and pyrethroid insecticides.

**Pediculicides**

- Malathion
- Carbaryl
- Synthetic pyrethroids:
  — permethrin
  — phenothrin

Preparations with an aqueous basis are less likely than those with an alcohol basis to irritate an excoriated scalp, they do not irritate the bronchi of people with asthma, and they are not flammable. None of these insecticides is fully ovicidal, and treatment should therefore be repeated after 7–10 days in order to kill any louse nymphs emerging from surviving eggs.

A new approach to topical treatment is the introduction of agents with a mode of action that is essentially to asphyxiate lice, such as dimeticone. An advantage of these is that there is little potential for the development of resistance.

Several over-the-counter head louse treatments contain tea-tree or lavender oil, and there is anecdotal evidence that they are effective. However, they have not been formally assessed in clinical trials.

A simple physical method of treatment involves washing the hair with an ordinary shampoo followed by the application of generous quantities of conditioner. The hair is then combed with a fine-toothed comb with closely set teeth, which removes any lice. This process is repeated every 4 days for 2 weeks.

## Clothing lice (*Pediculus humanus*)

*The louse*
*Has very little 'nous',*
*Its only pursuit*
*Is the hirsute.*

*I. Kenvyn Evans*

The clothing or body louse is a parasite that thrives in association with poverty and poor hygiene. It lives on, and lays its eggs in the seams of, clothing, and only moves on to the body to feed on blood. It is still common in the poorer countries of the world, but in an affluent society its usual hosts are down-and-outs and vagrants who have only one set of clothes that are never removed or cleaned. An individual who regularly changes clothing and maintains a reasonable standard of hygiene will never harbour clothing lice because the lice do not survive laundering and ironing of garments. Clothing lice are vectors of epidemic typhus, a rickettsial disease that has been responsible for millions of deaths over the centuries.

## Clinical features

Clothing lice usually provoke itching, and their host is often covered in excoriations. The itching appears to be the result of an acquired hypersensitivity to louse salivary antigens. If clothing louse infection is suspected there is no point in searching the patient for lice—you may be lucky and find an occasional louse at lunch on the body, but it is the clothing you should examine (Figure 5.8).

Figure 5.8 Clothing lice and eggs residing in a sock.

## Treatment

All the patient requires is a bath. A complete change of clean clothing should be supplied and the infested clothing either destroyed or laundered at temperatures of 60°C or above. Dry cleaning or use of a tumble drier is an alternative.

## Crab lice (*Phthirus pubis*)

> *It's no good standing on the seat*
> *The crabs in here can jump 10 feet.*
> *If you think that's rather high,*
> *Go next door, the buggers fly!*
>
> *Toilet graffito*

Crab lice, also known as pubic lice and love bugs, and in France as *papillons d'amour*, are usually transmitted during close physical contact with an infected individual, in spite of the above allegation of contagion from toilet seats. At one time they were thought to be rather sedentary lice, but experiments subsequently demonstrated that when its host is sleeping the crab louse becomes quite active. It is a louse adapted to living in hair of a particular density. It cannot colonize scalp hair, except at the margins of the scalp, but pubic, axillary, beard and eyelash hair are perfectly acceptable to it, and in an extremely hairy male most of the body may be teeming with lice. The crab louse is so named because of its squat shape and powerful claws, resembling a crab's pincers (Figure 5.9), with which it grasps hair. Female crab lice, similar to head lice, stick their eggs to hair shafts with a cement material.

## Clinical features

Itching, usually nocturnal, is the symptom that draws the host's attention to these little passengers. Self-examination then reveals the reason for the itch, and the doctor is often presented with a folded piece of paper containing 'specimens'. When folded paper is opened it has a tendency to flick its contents in all directions, leaving the unlucky recipient anxiously awaiting signs of personal contamination for weeks thereafter.

Lice are usually visible on the affected areas, but sometimes their eggs, which are a brown colour, are easier to see. If the parasites are very numerous the underclothes may be speckled with spots of altered blood excreted by the lice. Lice on the eyelids festoon the lashes with their eggs (Figure 5.10). Children may acquire crab lice as a result of normal close physical contact with an infected parent. The lice will colonize the eyelashes and scalp margin. As an isolated finding, crab louse infection in a child should not be considered indicative of sexual abuse.

## Treatment

The same pediculicides that are used to eradicate head lice are effective against crab lice, but aqueous preparations should be used because alcohol basis preparations will irritate the scrotum. The whole body should be treated, including the scalp if there is evidence of lice on the scalp margins. Sexual contacts should also be treated.

Figure 5.9 The crab louse.

3x

Figure 5.10 Crab louse eggs on the eyelashes.

The treatment should be repeated after an interval of 7–10 days.

Eyelash infection may be treated by the application of white soft paraffin (Vaseline) three times a day for 2–3 weeks. This acts by blocking the louse respiratory system, thereby suffocating the insects.

# Papular urticaria

Often referred to as 'heat bumps' by patients, papular urticaria is a typical response to the bites of a number of arthropods, including biting flies, mosquitoes, mites, fleas and bed bugs. The lesions are small urticated papules (Figure 5.11), usually grouped (sometimes in groups of three, fancifully labelled 'breakfast, lunch and dinner'), and they may be surmounted by a tiny vesicle. They are so itchy that their tops are rapidly excoriated. They develop as a result of a hypersensitivity response to antigens in the arthropods' saliva. Eventually, in many people, immunological tolerance to the antigens develops and they subsequently do not react to the bites.

## Fleas

*May the fleas of a thousand camels infest your armpits!*

*Arab curse*

The most common cause of papular urticaria acquired in the home environment is flea bites. It is not the human flea, *Pulex irritans*, that is

Figure 5.11 Papular urticaria.

responsible, but fleas with natural hosts of household pets. A familiar clinical picture is of multiple lesions, some of which may form blisters, around the ankles of women (Figure 5.12). Men are rarely

Figure 5.12 Flea bites on the ankles.

Figure 5.13 A cat flea.

affected, because socks and trousers deny fleas access to the ankles.

Cats and dogs are perambulating quadripedal 'meals-on-wheels' for the fleas (Figure 5.13). However, although fleas are present on the animals, their numbers are small in comparison with the fleas in various stages of development scattered throughout the household. Flea eggs are not sticky, and when laid by fleas feeding on an animal they drop out of the coat into the surroundings—the cat-basket, the carpet, the sofa or the counterpane. Eggs, larvae, pupae and adult fleas are present in all these areas. Hence, the house should be treated, as well as the pets. There are commercially available preparations designed to be sprayed around the house on carpets and soft furnishings, and veterinary products to be applied topically or fed to the animal, usually containing synthetic equivalents of insect growth regulatory hormones that interfere with flea development.

Occasionally, bird fleas will gain access to homes from nests under the eaves, and may be responsible for more extensive lesions of papular urticaria.

## Bed bugs (*Cimex lectularius*)

> The butterfly has wings of gold,
> The firefly wings of flame,
> The bed bug has no wings at all,
> But he gets there just the same.

Perhaps this rhyme relates to the, probably inaccurate, tale that if one attempts to stop bed bugs crawling up bed legs at night by placing the legs in bowls of water, the cunning bugs climb the walls, cross the ceiling, and drop on the occupants of the bed from above.

Bed bugs are not the most appealing of creatures. They live in dilapidated housing behind peeling wallpaper and rotten skirting boards, and emerge during the night to feed on the sleeping occupants of bedrooms. They feed on blood and, although the process of feeding does not cause the host any pain, a reaction to the bites of the bugs usually results in papular urticaria or bullous lesions. These insects are 5–6 mm long, dark brown in colour and can move quite rapidly. Although bed-bug infestation of houses in developed countries is uncommon, there has been an increase in reported cases in recent years—thought to be related to resistance to insecticides and transport of the bugs in the luggage of travellers returning from parts of the world where they are common. If infestation is suspected, pest control agencies should be employed to inspect and disinfest the building.

## Animal mites

Human contact with animals with sarcoptic mange may result in the development of scattered itchy papules, often on areas coming into contact with the animals, e.g. the abdomen and thighs if a mangy dog sits on its owner's lap. It is highly unlikely that these animal mites will establish themselves on humans, because they are species specific, but there have been a few reports in which it is said to have occurred.

Dogs, cats and rabbits are the natural hosts of mites of the genus *Cheyletiella*, and these may cause skin lesions in humans. Dogs are the usual culprits. On the animal, the mites provoke a heavy scurf over the back (known in veterinary circles as 'walking dandruff'), but hardly bother it otherwise. On the owner, itchy papules appear, principally on the abdomen, but occasionally also on the thighs and arms—sites of contact with the animal. The diagnosis can be confirmed by taking combings from the animal's coat and demonstrating the mite microscopically. Once the animal has been treated by a veterinary practitioner, the human skin lesions resolve spontaneously.

Bird mites may gain access to houses from nests under the eaves, and can cause itchy papular lesions.

## Ticks

Ixodid, or hard ticks, are very common, particularly in wooded areas where there are deer populations. They feed on blood, and their barbed mouthparts are held in the skin of the host during feeding by a protein cement material. If a tick is pulled off the skin abruptly, its mouthparts may be left *in situ*, and will provoke a foreign-body reaction.

Ixodid ticks are vectors of Lyme disease which is caused by the spirochaete *Borrelia burgdorferi*. Lyme disease (named after the town in Connecticut where its association with ticks was first discovered) affects the skin, joints, central nervous system and heart. In the early stages, oral therapy with amoxicillin or doxycycline for 3 weeks is recommended. In the later stages, with bacterial dissemination, treatment with intravenous ceftriaxone or cefotaxime is required.

Probably the best way to remove a tick is to grasp it as close to the skin as possible with fine tweezers or forceps, and exert gentle continuous traction.

# 6

# Acne, acneiform eruptions and rosacea

*Out, damned spot! Out, I say!*
*Shakespeare,* Macbeth v.i

## Introduction

This chapter deals with disorders that cause papules and pustules, often known in the vernacular as 'spots' or 'zits'. Some are aetiologically related and can properly be called variants of acne (a corruption of the Greek *akme*—a point). Others produce lesions closely or superficially resembling 'true' acne: the acneiform disorders and rosacea. A summary of the 'acne family' is given below.

---

**The acne family**

**Acne vulgaris**
- 'Classical'
- Infantile and juvenile onset
- Late onset
- Severe (acne conglobata, nodulocystic)
- With systemic symptoms (acne fulminans)

**Secondary acne**
- Endocrine associated
- Medicaments
- Oils
- Chloracne

**Hidradenitis suppurativa**

---

*Lecture Notes: Dermatology,* 10th edition. © RAC Graham-Brown and DA Burns. Published 2011 by Blackwell Publishing Ltd.

# Acne vulgaris and its variants

## Acne vulgaris

About 80% of people develop some spottiness. Acne may be very mild indeed, but, at its most severe, it can cause gross and unsightly changes.

Acne may be associated with underlying endocrinological abnormalities (see below) but this is rare.

## Age of onset and course

The first problems are usually encountered in adolescence, although there are exceptions (see below).

Lesions of acne vary considerably over time, most patients noticing fluctuations in the number and severity of spots. In girls this is often related to the menstrual cycle. The condition frequently deteriorates at times of stress.

Acne usually gets generally worse for a while before gradually settling after 2–3 years, and usually disappearing altogether. The peak of severity is earlier in girls than in boys. In some individuals, the time course may be much more prolonged, with lesions continuing to develop well into adult life.

There are two groups, described below, in whom true acne develops outside adolescence.

### Infantile/juvenile acne

Typical acne is occasionally seen in infants and children (especially boys), usually at 3–12 months of age. Although lesions subside after 4–5 years, adolescence often heralds a severe recrudescence. Endocrine abnormalities are very rare, but should be considered, especially in a girl with signs of virilism.

### Late-onset acne

A number of women and some men develop acne in their 20s and beyond. In women, this is often with marked premenstrual exacerbations. Polycystic ovary syndrome should be excluded, but endocrinological investigation is otherwise usually unremarkable.

## The psychological impact of acne

Acne can make life miserable, and its predilection for the teens and 20s means that it affects those least well equipped to cope.

The face is prominently involved which, in adolescence, assumes increasing importance as self-image develops. At the time when acne strikes, major relationships outside the family and close circles of same-sex friends are becoming increasingly crucial. However, the psychological impact of acne is by no means always related to the degree of severity as perceived by an outsider. People often spend just as long staring miserably into the mirror when there are only a few spots as when there are hundreds.

## Clinical features

### Physical signs

Acne has a characteristic distribution.

Figure 6.1 This girl's face shows the typical greasy skin of the acne sufferer, in addition to papules and pustules.

## The appearance of the skin

The first physical sign to note is that the face and upper trunk become very greasy (Figure 6.1) due to increased production of sebum. This is normal at puberty, but is excessive in those with acne. Scalp hair is often very greasy too. Greasiness alone may be bad enough for patients to seek advice.

## The individual lesions of acne

A cardinal feature is that there are several different types of lesion at any one time.

---

**Site and distribution of acne**

- Face, any part of which may be involved
- Neck, especially posteriorly
- Ears
- Upper back
- Anterior chest, in 'V' from the shoulders to the xiphisternum
- Shoulders

---

**Acne vulgaris lesions**

- Comedones:
  — closed ('whiteheads')
  — open ('blackheads')
- Papules
- Pustules
- Nodules
- Cysts
- Scars

---

In severe acne, lesions may extend down the arms, across the whole of the central back, and on to the buttocks.

### Comedones (singular: comedo)

The presence of comedones is a key diagnostic aid, because they are really seen in acne only in young people. There are two types: closed (or 'whitehead') and open (or 'blackhead').

Figure 6.2 Closed comedones.

Closed comedones are more easily felt than seen. They are very small papules, with a central point or elevation (Figure 6.2). They are often most numerous on the forehead and cheeks. There is little or no inflammation.

Open comedones (blackheads) are dilated blocked hair follicles, but it is not clear what causes the characteristic black dots. Burnt-out inflammatory lesions may leave multiheaded blackheads, particularly on the shoulders and upper trunk. Blackheads are virtually pathognomonic of acne in the younger patient (although advanced solar damage may cause them).

### Papules and pustules

The majority of patients with acne develop papules and pustules, often on a red base. They may itch or be quite painful. Papules develop rapidly, sometimes over only a few hours, and frequently become pustular as they evolve. They resolve over the course of a few days. New lesions may arise in exactly the same site on many occasions.

### Nodules and cysts

With increasing severity, and as the inflammation extends deeper, the size of visible and palpable lesions increases, resulting in deep-seated nodules and cysts (Figures 6.3 and 6.4). Many patients develop a few, but some have large numbers: a situation for which the term 'acne conglobata' is used.

Such lesions are often extremely uncomfortable and last much longer than more superficial changes. Some become chronic, and may result in permanent cyst formation (see Chapter 9).

Figure 6.3 Acne conglobata.

Figure 6.4 Severe acne on the back.

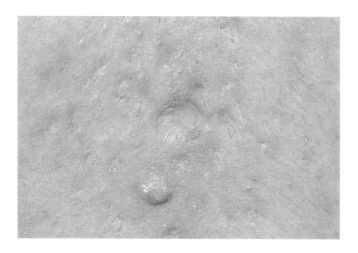

Figure 6.5 Atrophic scarring in acne.

## Scars

The final common pathway for the inflammatory process of acne is scarring, which will remain as a lifetime's legacy of adolescent anguish. Characteristically, small, deep, 'ice-pick' scars occur, but more severe disease can leave gross changes, with atrophy (Figure 6.5) or keloid formation (see Chapter 9).

## Systemic symptoms (acne fulminans)

Very occasionally a young man (almost always) develops severe nodulocystic acne accompanied by fever, malaise, and joint pain and swelling. This is known as 'acne fulminans'.

## Pathogenesis of acne

The aetiopathology of acne remains to be elucidated fully. However, several key factors probably contribute to the final picture (Figure 6.6), although we cannot fully explain every aspect of the disorder: the occurrence of prepubertal acne, for example.

As the inflammation subsides, a variable amount of fibrosis occurs, which may produce scarring, particularly with repeated episodes at the same site. Sometimes epithelial remnants become walled off by fibrosis, producing cysts.

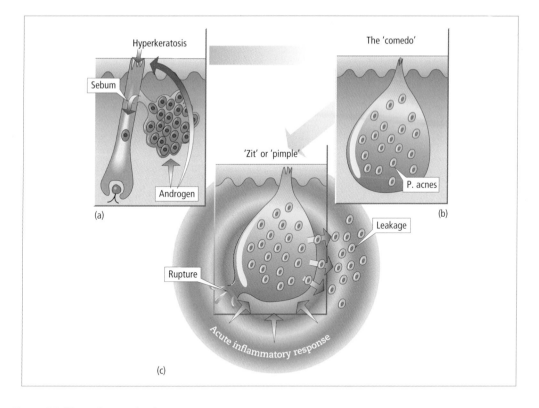

Figure 6.6 The pathogenesis of acne.

## Pathogenesis of acne

1 Androgens (usually in normal amounts) stimulate increased sebum production

2 Hair follicles with particularly large sebaceous glands (on the face, neck, chest and back) become blocked by hyperkeratosis

3 This results in the closed comedo

4 Within the follicle, an obligate anaerobe (*Propionibacterium acnes*) proliferates

5 This organism acts on sebum, releasing inflammatory chemicals

6 These leak into the surrounding dermis

7 The body mounts an intense acute inflammatory response, the result of which is the papule, pustule or nodule

## Treatment of acne

### Topical therapies

Many over-the-counter remedies simply make the skin flaky and unblock hair follicles (e.g. sulfur and other astringents).

Topical antiseptics are often prescribed, but are of little value.

Benzoyl peroxide is widely used. It definitely reduces the number of comedones but must be used regularly and over a sustained period. There are several concentrations: start with a weaker preparation, applied once daily, and gradually progress to higher strengths.

Vitamin A derivatives (retinoids) also reduce comedones. Preparations in this category include retinoic acid, isotretinoin (13-*cis*-retinoic acid) and adapalene. All may help but can be irritant.

Topical antibiotics (especially tetracyclines, erythromycin and clindamycin) are generally applied once daily. All have been shown to be useful in milder acne. However, resistance of *P. acnes* to topical antibiotics is a problem. Some preparations combine antibiotics with other agents such as benzoyl peroxide.

---

**Treatments for acne**

**Topical**
- Benzoyl peroxide
- Retinoids
- Sulfur and astringents
- Topical antiseptics, antibiotics and combination products

**Systemic**
- Antibiotics
- Cyproterone acetate
- 13-*cis*-Retinoic acid (isotretinoin)
- Steroids

**Surgical intervention**

---

## Systemic therapies

Antibiotics are the mainstay of the treatment of papulopustular acne in primary care in the UK. They reduce bacterial counts, at least initially, but also have direct anti-inflammatory effects.

The most effective are the tetracyclines, erythromycin and trimethoprim. To work, antibiotics must be fat soluble, so penicillins are useless. Most tetracyclines should be taken on an empty stomach. Tetracyclines are contraindicated in children aged <12, and in pregnant or lactating women.

Cyproterone acetate is an antiandrogen that can be given only to women. It is given along with oestrogen (as co-cyprindiol) to prevent menorrhagia and to ensure contraceptive cover (as it feminizes a male fetus). Its effect is rather slow.

13-*cis*-Retinoic acid (isotretinoin) is a highly effective oral vitamin A derivative that dramatically reduces sebum production. It is the first choice in UK secondary care, because it is available only on hospital prescription. Over 90% of patients have complete clearance and in up to 80% there is no relapse. There are several side effects:

## Side effects of isotretinoin

- Dry skin, lips and eyes
- Dry nasal mucosae with epistaxes
- Mild alopecia
- Generalised arthralgia and myalgia
- Raised blood fat levels
- Altered liver function tests
- Teratogenicity
- Possible psychological disturbances

The most serious problem with isotretinoin is that significant fetal abnormalities are very common. All female patients must therefore be advised not to get pregnant and should be monitored very carefully throughout treatment. In the UK clinicians and patients should adhere to an agreed 'pregnancy prevention protocol'. The drug has developed a reputation for causing psychological disturbances. Whether this is a significant causal effect remains controversial, but all patients should be warned about mood changes, especially depression.

Dapsone may also be a useful addition in patients with very troublesome acne, and is safe.

Steroids can be used intralesionally or systemically in severe acne (they are virtually always needed in acne fulminans).

## Surgical intervention

Simple measures, such as using a comedone extractor on multiple comedones, may improve the appearance. It certainly gives great pleasure and satisfaction to a mother, or a girl- or boyfriend who likes to pop out blackheads! Large, residual cysts may need to be excised, but there is a risk of keloid scarring. Plastic and dermatological surgeons can sometimes help acne scarring with superficial laser therapy or dermabrasion, but this must not be attempted until the acne is fully under control.

## Management of a patient with acne

The approach to treatment must be tailored to the individual, but there are some helpful guidelines. Let's first dispel some myths!

## Assessment of the patient

It is useful to consider acne in three broad severity bands: mild, moderate and severe.

### Mild acne

This may respond to topical treatment alone. Begin with benzoyl peroxide, retinoic acid, isotretinoin or adapalene, and/or a topical antibiotic. An antibiotic/benzoyl peroxide combination can be a useful option.

### Moderate acne

This should initially be treated with a combination of a topical agent and oral oxytetracycline or erythromycin (either of these in a dose of 500 mg twice daily), continuing for at least 3–6 months before reassessing. Alternative tetracyclines (doxycycline, lymecycline, minocycline) have their advocates: usually on the basis of better absorption or tolerance.

If the response is not satisfactory, or if the changes are severe at the outset, acne should be managed as outlined below.

### Severe acne

Girls may respond to cyproterone acetate (co-cyprindiol) with or without antibiotics, allowing at least 6 months for a response. Dapsone at a dose of 25 mg twice daily can be helpful.

However, many girls and most young men with severe or persistent acne eventually require isotretinoin, usually for 4–6 months. The daily dose may begin at 0.5 mg/kg but may need to be raised to 1 mg/kg. We have already stressed the need for counselling and surveillance in females, but liver function and lipids should also be monitored.

Intralesional steroids are useful for acute inflammatory lesions. Very rarely, systemic steroid therapy may be required, especially in acne fulminans.

Surgical intervention may be required later to help overcome the devastation wreaked by this degree of acne.

**Acne assessment**

**Mild**

- Only comedones *and/or* only a few papulopustular lesions restricted to the face

**Moderate**

- More papulopustular lesions on the face or over a wider area *and/or* occasional nodules

**Severe**

- Very widespread papulopustular lesions *and/or* nodulocystic lesions *and/or* systemic symptoms

*or* acne of moderate severity, failing to settle within 6 months of therapy

*or* acne of whatever severity with significant psychological upset

# Secondary acne

Acne lesions may arise as a consequence of other primary pathological processes. Such 'secondary' acne is often monomorphic and generally mild.

An exception is acne occurring in patients with endocrine abnormalities. The most common is polycystic ovary syndrome, in which acne of any severity may accompany hirsutism, menstrual irregularities and infertility. Any cause of abnormally high circulating androgen levels (such as tumours) may result in bad acne, whereas lesions in Cushing's syndrome are milder.

Topical preparations (including medicaments) such as greasy ointments, pomades and topical steroids may induce comedones and papules, particularly on the face. Several drugs induce acneiform lesions or make pre-existing acne worse, notably systemic steroids, phenytoin, isoniazid and lithium.

Oil-induced acne occurs when mineral oils come into close contact with the skin. This is often at unusual sites, such as the lower abdomen and thighs.

Chloracne is a specific change in which comedones appear after exposure to chlorinated chemical compounds. Famous examples are the release of dioxin from an explosion at Seveso in Italy and the poisoning of a prominent Ukrainian politician. Systemic upsets also occur.

## Hidradenitis suppurativa

Although uncommon, this distinctive disorder results in very unpleasant, chronic, relapsing sepsis in the apocrine areas of the axillae and groins (Figure 6.7). Many apocrine glands open into the upper part of pilosebaceous follicles and comedonal occlusion of the ducts may be the initial event in hidradenitis.

Recurrent painful abscesses and sinus tracks develop. Many patients with hidradenitis have concurrent severe acne, or have had acne in the past.

Some patients improve on long-term antibiotics (including agents with activity against anaerobic bacteria), antiandrogens and/or isotretinoin, but many require plastic surgery.

(a)

(b)

Figure 6.7 Hidradenitis suppurativa of (a) axilla and (b) groin.

## Acneiform disorders

Several conditions mimic acne, but close examination will reveal important differences.

Pseudofolliculitis barbae (shaving rash): produces small papules in the beard area and is more common in those with naturally curly hair, especially African–Caribbean individuals. Occasionally small keloids develop. The process may involve the nape of the neck, when it is usually termed 'acne keloidalis'. Treatment is unsatisfactory.

Acne excoriée (*des jeunes filles*) is typically seen in teenage girls who present with facial excoriations but very few primary lesions. There are no comedones. This is a form of neurotic excoriation (see Chapter 20), and patients need to be given a clear explanation and helped to try and reduce the self-inflicted damage.

Pityrosporum folliculitis, caused by *Malassezia* sp., features follicular papules and pustules on the trunk, without other features of acne. The condition responds to antifungal agents such as miconazole.

In keratosis pilaris, small spiky projections develop at the mouth of hair follicles, especially on the upper, outer arms and shoulders. Lesions may appear on the face, especially in children, and are occasionally pustular. A family history is common. Topical retinoic acid may be helpful.

Rosacea is an important differential diagnosis of acne, and is sometimes erroneously called 'acne rosacea'. It occurs in both sexes, but most frequently affects middle-aged women. The sites of predilection are the central cheeks, forehead and glabellar region, end of the nose and chin (Figure

Figure 6.8 Rosacea: (a) showing typical distribution and (b) inflammatory papules and pustules.

Figure 6.9 Rhinophyma.

6.8). The eruption consists of small papules and pustules arising in crops on an erythematous, telangiectatic background.

There are no comedones. Patients frequently complain of flushing easily with heat or alcohol, and migraines are more common. In men, severe involvement of the nose leads to marked sebaceous hyperplasia known as rhinophyma (Figure 6.9).

The treatment of choice is tetracyclines, given for several weeks in similar doses to those for moderate acne (see above). Topical metronidazole is also effective and often combined with oral therapy. It may be possible to tail off the treatment, but the condition often recurs. Topical steroids make matters worse. Rhinophyma is best dealt with by plastic surgeons. Severe resistant rosacea may respond to oral isotretinoin.

Perioral dermatitis (note for classical purists: it should really be '*circum*-oral' [Latin] or 'peristomal' [Greek]) produces a clinical appearance somewhat reminiscent of rosacea (see Figure 22.3). It is often associated with topical steroid abuse. (For more details see Chapter 22.)

# 7

# Eczema

The terms 'eczema' (Greek, meaning 'to boil over') and 'dermatitis' are synonymous. 'Atopic eczema' is therefore the same as 'atopic dermatitis', and 'seborrhoeic eczema' and 'seborrhoeic dermatitis' are the same. Eczema/dermatitis is a type of inflammatory reaction pattern in the skin that may be provoked by a number of external or internal factors.

## Clinical features

The principal symptom of eczema is itching. The clinical signs depend on its aetiology, site and duration, but usually comprise erythema, oedema, papules, vesicles and exudation (Figure 7.1). An acute eczema will have all these features, and might also have a bullous component. In a chronic eczema oedema is not a prominent feature, but the epidermis becomes thickened and the skin surface markings are exaggerated (lichenification) (Figure 7.2). A common feature of eczema of the hands or feet is the formation of painful fissures in the skin overlying joints.

A phenomenon that is seen with an acute dermatitis, particularly allergic contact dermatitis, is secondary spread of the eczema to sites distant from the originally affected area. Occasionally, most of the body surface is affected, and eczema is one cause of generalized exfoliative dermatitis.

Other changes in the skin that may accompany eczema include scratch marks and secondary bacterial infection. Prolonged scratching and rubbing of the skin tend to polish fingernails, and patients with chronic eczema often have nails that look as if they have a coat of clear nail varnish.

*Lecture Notes: Dermatology*, 10th edition. © RAC Graham-Brown and DA Burns. Published 2011 by Blackwell Publishing Ltd.

## Classification

We still have a great deal to learn about the aetiology of certain types of eczema, so any attempt at classification is based on our present state of ignorance. A commonly employed system of classification divides cases of eczema into 'exogenous', where an external agent is responsible, and 'endogenous', where the problem is principally constitutional. There are, however, frequent cases in which more than one factor may be operating, e.g. the hairdresser with hand dermatitis who has atopic dermatitis and also superimposed irritant dermatitis from contact with shampoos. Do not be too rigid in your attempts to classify a particular dermatitis— it may not fit a recognized category, and it might be preferable to use a more general term such as 'probably endogenous'. The classification in the box includes most of the types of eczema you are likely to encounter.

---

### Eczema classification

**Exogenous**
- Primary irritant contact dermatitis
- Allergic contact dermatitis

**Endogenous**
- Atopic eczema
- Seborrhoeic dermatitis
- Discoid eczema
- Varicose eczema
- Endogenous eczema of the palms and soles
- Asteatotic eczema (eczema craquelé)

Figure 7.1 Typical eczema.

Figure 7.2 Lichenified eczema.

# Exogenous eczema

## Primary irritant dermatitis

Primary irritants physically damage the skin, and include acids, alkalis, detergents and petroleum products. Some strong irritants will produce an immediate effect, whereas with weaker irritants the effects are cumulative. Anyone who has atopic dermatitis is more susceptible to the effects of primary irritants. The housewife with a 'couch-potato' husband, eight children and no washing machine or dishwasher is a good candidate for a cumulative primary irritant dermatitis, because her hands will be perpetually immersed in washing-up liquid and soap powder. However, the wife of a merchant banker with 2.2 children, a nanny and a kitchen full of modern appliances is hardly likely to inconvenience her epidermis to the same degree. The typical appearance of house-wives' hand dermatitis is dryness of the palms and fingertips, often with painful fissures in the skin creases and on the finger pulps.

Occupational irritant dermatitis is common, e.g. hairdressing apprentices may spend a sub-stantial part of the day with their hands immersed in shampoo on their clients' heads, and many develop irritant dermatitis. If they also have atopic eczema their hand problem often becomes so severe that they are forced to leave hairdressing. A similar situation is seen in machine-tool operators whose hands are immersed in cutting fluid (Figure 7.3). It follows that young people with atopic der-matitis should be advised to avoid careers in occu-pations involving contact with irritants, such as hairdressing, engineering, vehicle mechanics, nursing and catering.

In theory, the treatment is simple—either remove the patient from contact with the irritant or protect the hands against it. In practice it is often impossible to avoid contact with the irritant without changing jobs, and in many occupations the nature of the work means that wearing gloves is impracticable. The skin can be helped to a certain extent by the liberal use of emollients (see Chapter 22), but it cannot be restored to normal while exposure to irritants continues. What usually happens is that severe dermatitis eventually forces a change of occupation, or individuals with milder problems learn to tolerate them.

**Figure 7.3** Hand dermatitis in a machine-tool operator.

## Allergic contact dermatitis

This is due to a delayed hypersensitivity reaction to an external allergen. There are innumerable chemicals that can act as allergens, but most rarely cause problems. Some chemicals are such potent allergens that a single exposure will cause sensitization, but many require multiple exposures before sensitization occurs. It is possible to be exposed to an allergen for years, and then suddenly develop hypersensitivity.

Frequent causes of contact dermatitis include nickel, colophony, rubber additives, chromate, hair dyes and topical medicaments—both their active ingredients and components of their bases.

## Nickel dermatitis

Nickel is the most common cause of contact dermatitis in women, whereas contact allergy to nickel is uncommon in men. Sensitization to nickel usually occurs in childhood and early adult life as a result of ear piercing and the wearing of cheap costume jewellery. The problem usually begins with itchy earlobes, but it is dermatitis caused by the metallic components of other garments that brings the nickel-sensitive patient to the dermatologist. In the pre-miniskirt era, suspender dermatitis was the most common presentation of nickel sensitivity. Suspender belts were perhaps more functional than decorative in those days, and the bare metal clips produced patches of dermatitis on the thighs. With the advent of the miniskirt and tights, suspender dermatitis disappeared from the dermatology clinic. In more recent times it is the jeans stud that has become an important source of nickel, and a patch of eczema adjacent to the umbilicus is virtually pathognomonic of nickel sensitivity (Figure 7.4).

If nickel dermatitis is suspected, look at the skin on the earlobes and wrists. In spite of being aware that costume jewellery provokes a skin reaction, many women continue to wear a favourite pair of earrings from time to time, and will have dermatitis on the ears. Nickel dermatitis on the wrists is usually caused by the metal buckle on a watch strap. Stainless steel in wrist watches does not cause any problems because, although steel contains nickel, it is tightly bound and does not leach out.

The multitude of folk who have adopted the 'fashion' of having their delicate bodily parts pierced are perhaps fortunate in that the various rings and barbells dangling and protruding from them are made of good quality steel, and do not usually provoke dermatitis unless further embellished with costume jewellery. Anyone who is allergic to nickel should be advised to avoid costume jewellery (unless it is known to be nickel free), bare metal clips on underwear, metal buckles on shoes and metal zips. The metal stud on the front of jeans can be replaced by a button, and problems from watches can usually be avoided by wearing a Swatch watch, as the only metal in contact with the skin is the stainless steel battery compartment.

## Colophony

This is a resin that is a component of some adhesive plasters.

Figure 7.4 Contact dermatitis to nickel in jeans stud.

## Rubber dermatitis

During the manufacture of rubber, chemicals are used to speed up the vulcanization process (accelerators) and to prevent its oxidation (antioxidants), and these can cause allergic contact dermatitis.

In recent years there has been a marked increase in the occurrence of reactions to natural rubber latex protein in latex gloves. Latex protein can provoke an immediate hypersensitivity response, and reactions range from contact urticaria to rhinitis, asthma and anaphylaxis. Individuals affected are most often healthcare workers who frequently wear latex gloves, but patients who have undergone multiple procedures, most notably people with spina bifida, may also be affected. A significant factor contributing to this problem appears to have been that the demand for latex gloves outstripped supply, and some manufacturers subsequently produced gloves containing large amounts of free latex protein. This situation has been remedied, and it is hoped that latex allergy will now become less of a problem.

## Chromate

Chromium compounds have a number of industrial applications. They are also used in leather tanning, and are the major sensitizer in cement. Cement dermatitis is common in building workers.

## Hair dye dermatitis

Contact sensitivity to hair dye usually presents as severe dermatitis affecting the face, ears and scalp margin. Hair dyes are also a cause of contact dermatitis on the hands of hairdressers. The chemical usually responsible for hair dye dermatitis, paraphenylenediamine (PPD), is also sometimes mixed with henna and used in temporary tattoos, a form of decoration that is currently quite popular, and this may be responsible for severe allergic contact dermatitis.

## Topical medicaments

Medicament dermatitis is relatively common in dermatological practice, but perhaps not as common as might be expected if one considers the huge quantities of creams, lotions and potions used in the average household. Open any bathroom cabinet or bedside drawer in any house in the land and you will find creams for dry skin, creams for haemorrhoids, preparations for cuts and grazes, creams for insect bites and stings, and almost invariably a tube of a topical steroid.

Common causes of contact dermatitis in topical medicaments include antibiotics, particularly neomycin, local anaesthetics (except lidocaine, which is a rare sensitizer), antihistamines and preservatives. Dermatoses in which contact sensitivity to some of these agents may be a complicating factor include otitis externa, pruritus ani and venous leg ulcers. In recent years, contact allergy to topical steroids has emerged as a problem. It is usually discovered in patients who fail to respond or experience a deterioration in their skin condition while undergoing treatment with topical steroids.

## Occupational contact dermatitis

If occupational factors are thought to be responsible for contact dermatitis, a detailed history, including precise information about the nature of an individual's work, is essential. This should include not only information about present occupation but also details of previous employment. A history of significant improvement of the dermatitis during holiday periods is typical of a work-related dermatosis. If someone tells you that he was a 'saggar-maker's bottom knocker', enquire as to the nature of this exotic-sounding occupation (it used to be encountered in areas where ceramic ware was produced)—it is common to encounter terminology that is specific to a certain occupation, and is incomprehensible to those outside the trade. Establish what materials are handled at work, and if there have been any changes which coincided with the onset of the dermatitis. It is also useful to know if any workmates have the same problem. Seeing a patient in the working environment is often important in determining the cause of a dermatitis.

## Plant dermatitis

Plant dermatitis is relatively uncommon in Europe. In the past, reactions to household plants usually involved *Primula obconica,* and were caused by the allergen primin, but this has become less common with the introduction of allergen-free cultivars. Garden plants can also cause problems, and in summer exposure to the sap of certain plants and sunlight can provoke a so-called phytophotodermatitis—giant hogweed and other Umbelliferae are often implicated. A well-recognized scenario is the occurrence of a spattered blistering eruption in someone who, stripped to the waist in strong sunshine, has used a strimmer on weeds such as cow parsley (strimmer's dermatitis). Chrysanthemums also cause dermatitis, sesquiterpene lactones being the responsible allergens. The handling of garlic and tulip bulbs is a cause of fingertip dermatitis.

In the USA, the poison ivies (*Toxicodendron* spp.) are the most common cause of plant dermatitis, and in India feverfew (*Parthenium hysterophorus*) is the most troublesome.

Dermatitis caused by plants tends to present with a linear, vesiculobullous reaction on the exposed parts of the body.

## Diagnosis of allergic contact dermatitis

It is important to take a detailed history covering present occupation, previous occupations, hobbies and the use of topical medicaments. The distribution pattern of the dermatitis may suggest a possible allergen, and provoke further questions, e.g. eczema adjacent to the umbilicus prompts enquiry about previous problems with earrings. Certain patterns are characteristic of a particular allergen: in the days when 'strike anywhere' matches were in common use contact sensitivity to phosphorus sesquisulfide, which is present in the heads of the matches, was responsible for a combination of eczema on the face, in the ears, on the hands and on one or other thigh. The facial eczema was caused by contact with the smoke from the matches, the hand eczema by handling the matchbox, which had the chemical on the striking surface, and that on the thigh from carrying the box in a trouser pocket. The eczema in the ears was the result of using matches to clean them out!

However, when the cause is not as obvious it may require considerable detective work to track it down, and patch testing (see Chapter 2) is an essential component of the investigative process. Patch testing is quite different from prick or scratch testing. It is a delayed hypersensitivity response, in which the reaction takes 48h to develop, whereas prick or scratch tests elicit an immediate hypersensitivity response that develops within minutes. A standard battery of common allergens is used in routine patch testing, but other batteries of allergens, such as components of topical agents or occupational allergens, are also available. The majority of the allergens used are mixed in white soft paraffin to a specific concentration, because many are irritant in high concentration and might produce false-positive reactions. Patients sometimes claim that they are 'allergic' to materials that they use at work, and these may be presented to the dermatologist, often in unmarked jars. Such materials are often irritants, and should not be used for patch testing without obtaining further information about their constituents and potential toxicity, otherwise they might bore an untidy hole in the patient's back.

Positive reactions must be interpreted in the context of the patient's presenting problem—not all positives will be relevant.

Wait until an acute eczema has settled before patch testing—positive reactions may exacerbate the eczema.

## Treatment

Potent topical steroids (see Chapter 22) should be used to settle the eczema before patch testing. Once an allergen has been identified as the cause of a problem, the patient should be advised about its avoidance. If components of medicaments are involved, the patient's family doctor must be informed of what preparations the patient should avoid.

# Endogenous eczema

## Atopic eczema

The term 'atopy' implies a genetic predisposition to develop eczema, asthma and hay fever. A family history of atopy is common in patients with atopic eczema. Recently, it has been demonstrated that loss-of-function mutations in *FLG*, the gene encoding filaggrin (see Chapter 1) strongly predispose to atopic eczema. In addition, a greater prevalence of atopic eczema in developed 'westernized' countries than in developing countries, and evidence that the prevalence of atopic disease is increasing, are factors suggesting that environmental influences also play a part in pathogenesis. Other factors in its complex pathogenesis are immunological abnormalities and emotional influences. Immunological abnormalities in the atopic state include increased serum total IgE and specific IgE antibody to ingested or inhaled antigens (such as house-dust mite allergens), and preferential activation of the T-helper 2 (Th2) subset of CD4+ T cells, which produce interleukin 4 (IL-4), IL-5 and IL-13, all of which are involved in regulation of IgE synthesis by B lymphocytes. Staphylococci colonize the skin of patients with atopic eczema, and staphylococcal exotoxins with superantigen properties are also thought to play a pathogenic role.

Atopic eczema is not present at birth, but frequently appears in the first year of life. In early childhood the eczema is often generalized, but later a characteristic flexural involvement is seen—wrists, antecubital fossae, popliteal fossae and dorsa of feet (Figure 7.5). The skin is dry and intensely itchy. As a result of constant scratching and rubbing, the affected areas become thickened (lichenification). The course is typically punctuated by episodic exacerbations.

Atopic eczema often resolves in childhood, but may persist into adolescence and adult life, and there is no way of predicting the outcome. Those whose skin has apparently reverted to normal remain susceptible to the effects of primary irritants, which may provoke a recrudescence of eczema.

The most common complication is secondary bacterial infection, producing folliculitis or impetigo. Viral warts and molluscum contagiosum occur more frequently in atopic individuals, and herpes simplex infection may lead to

Figure 7.5 Flexural involvement in atopic eczema.

widespread skin lesions (see Chapter 3) and a severe illness (eczema herpeticum, Kaposi's varicelliform eruption).

## Treatment

An important aspect of the management of a child with atopic eczema is sympathetic explanation of the nature of the condition to his or her parents.

Emollients are essential in the management of the dry skin in atopic eczema. There are numerous emollients available, and it is often necessary to try a number of preparations in order to find one that is suitable for a particular individual. They can be used in combination at bath time, e.g. one as a soap substitute, a bath oil in the water and an emollient cream afterwards.

Topical steroids are invaluable in the treatment of atopic eczema. In young children mild steroids are the mainstay. In older children and adults more potent steroids are required, but the aim should always be to use the weakest preparation sufficient to control the disease. A topical steroid/antibacterial combination may be useful if eczema frequently becomes secondarily infected—obvious secondary infection should be treated with a systemic antibiotic such as flucloxacillin or erythromycin. Emollient/antimicrobial combinations may also be useful in reducing bacterial colonization of the skin.

In recent years, topical preparations of the calcineurin inhibitors tacrolimus and pimecrolimus have become available for the treatment of atopic eczema. An advantage of these products is that unlike topical steroids they do not produce skin atrophy. At present they are principally used in patients whose eczema has not responded to conventional therapy, and they can be particularly useful for facial eczema.

The wet-wrap technique is useful in the management of severe eczema, and medicated bandages such as zinc paste and ichthammol or zinc oxide and coal tar, applied over a topical steroid, are beneficial for eczema on the limbs. A sedative antihistamine at night may help to reduce scratching. Ultraviolet light treatment, either UVB or psoralens and UVA (PUVA therapy), helps some atopic individuals, but the eczema often relapses when treatment is stopped. Ciclosporin may be of great benefit to patients with severe atopic eczema.

The value of dietary manipulation is controversial. Some children appear to be helped by elimination diets in which dairy products, food additives, nuts and other foods suspected of exacerbating eczema are excluded, but in many there is no obvious benefit. Most dermatologists reserve dietary manipulation for severely affected children who fail to benefit from other treatment methods. It is dangerous to manipulate a child's diet without expert advice, because this can lead to nutritional deficiencies.

Figure 7.6 Seborrhoeic dermatitis.

Chinese herbal therapy is another controversial issue. Undoubtedly some individuals have benefited from Chinese herbal medicines, but there is concern about their potential for hepatotoxicity and nephrotoxicity, and some topical 'herbal' medicines have been shown to contain steroids.

## Seborrhoeic dermatitis

This is a constitutional disorder the exact pathogenesis of which is not fully understood, but in recent years the role of malassezia yeasts has been emphasized.

Seborrhoeic dermatitis affects the scalp, face, presternal area, upper back and flexures. Scalp involvement presents as itchy, diffuse scaling on an erythematous background. On the face, there is scaly erythema in the nasolabial folds and on the forehead, eyebrows and beard area (Figure 7.6). Lesions on the chest are often marginated. Flexural involvement produces a moist, glazed erythema. Particularly severe seborrhoeic dermatitis occurs in patients with AIDS.

Seborrhoeic dermatitis usually requires treatment over many years, as there is no cure for this condition. It is important to make this clear to patients, who otherwise tend to try many treatments in their quest for a permanent solution to the problem. Topical hydrocortisone is effective, but the problem recurs when treatment is stopped. Steroid lotions or gels and tar shampoos will help the scalp. Ketoconazole shampoo and cream, and imidazole/hydrocortisone combinations, are also effective.

## Discoid eczema

In this disorder, scattered, well-demarcated areas of exuding and crusting eczema develop on the trunk and limbs. A potent topical steroid is usually required to keep the condition controlled. Its aetiology is unknown.

## Varicose eczema (stasis dermatitis; gravitational eczema)

Chronic venous hypertension is frequently associated with eczematous changes on the legs. Secondary spread to the forearms may occur.

Mild or moderate potency topical steroids will usually suppress the eczema.

## Endogenous eczema of the palms and soles

Some patients develop a symmetrical pattern of eczema affecting the palms and soles that is chronic, and does not appear to be related to any external factors. Long-term treatment with potent topical steroids is usually required.

An episodic form of eczema of the palms and soles, in which bulla formation occurs, is known as acute pompholyx (Figure 7.7). This develops rapidly, and can be severely incapacitating. Secondary bacterial infection is common. It usually responds to treatment with potassium permanganate soaks and a systemic antibiotic such as flucloxacillin or erythromycin. The trigger for these episodes is unknown. Ciclosporin or the oral

Figure 7.7 Pompholyx.

Figure 7.8 Eczema craquelé.

retinoid alitretinoin may be of benefit in recalcitrant eczema of the palms.

## Asteatotic eczema

With increasing age, the lipid content of the stratum corneum decreases, and elderly skin is particularly susceptible to 'degreasing' agents. Asteatotic eczema (also known as eczema craquelé) is usually seen on the legs, but it may also occur on the lower abdomen and arms, and occasionally it is generalized. It is common in elderly patients admitted to hospital and bathed more frequently than they bathe at home. A crazy-paving pattern develops (Figure 7.8), and the skin itches. Treatment with an emollient is sometimes adequate, but a mild topical steroid ointment is often necessary.

## Juvenile plantar dermatosis

As its name suggests, this condition occurs in children. It is thought to be related to wearing training shoes and socks made of synthetic materials, and may represent a form of irritant dermatitis. It became prevalent in the 1970s when 'trainers' were introduced as footwear. The weight-bearing areas of the feet are dry and shiny, and painful fissures occur (Figure 7.9). Changing to cotton or woollen socks and leather shoes sometimes helps, as does the liberal use of emollients. Topical steroids are usually ineffective. It almost invariably resolves by the early teens.

We are of the impression that this condition is becoming less prevalent—possibly as a result of

Figure 7.9 Juvenile plantar dermatosis.

changes in the components of footwear, rather than a reduction in the number of individuals wearing training shoes.

# 8

# Psoriasis

*Dermatologists do it on a grand scale.*

Anon

## Introduction

Psoriasis is one of the most common and most important of the inflammatory dermatoses: up to 3% of the population of western countries, India and the Far East develop psoriasis during their lifetime. It is also common in parts of Africa. As most of those who develop psoriasis have lesions for the rest of their lives, it is clearly a considerable problem.

It is still not known why psoriasis develops when it does. There is undoubtedly a strong genetic component, particularly if the disease begins in youth or early adulthood. However, although a family history is common, there is often no clear-cut inheritance pattern. What does seem clear is that the cascade of changes described below probably results from an interaction between T cells and keratinocytes, with the involvement of various cytokines and chemoattractants—notably interleukins 1 and 8 (IL-1 and IL-8), tumour necrosis factor-$\alpha$ (TNF-$\alpha$), E-selectin and intercellular adhesion molecule-1 (ICAM-1).

Some well-recognized triggers may induce psoriasis in susceptible individuals, notably trauma

*Lecture Notes: Dermatology*, 10th edition. © RAC Graham-Brown and DA Burns. Published 2011 by Blackwell Publishing Ltd.

and infection. Some authorities also maintain that stress may induce or exacerbate the condition. However, there is no clear understanding of what causes some areas of skin to turn into plaques of psoriasis while others remain normal.

## Pathology

The pathological process is a combination of epidermal hyperproliferation and accumulation of inflammatory cells. The 'epidermal transit time' is markedly reduced from the normal 8–10 weeks to a few days. There is also increased vascularity of the upper dermis. Figure 8.1 provides a schematic representation of a psoriatic plaque. The cardinal features are given in the box.

---

**Cardinal features**

- Marked thickening of the epidermis (acanthosis)
- Absence of the granular cell layer
- Retention of nuclei in the horny layer (parakeratosis)
- Accumulations of polymorphs in the horny layer (microabscesses)
- Dilated capillary loops in the upper dermis

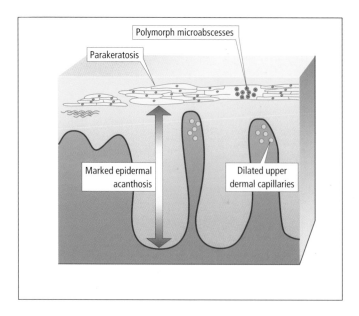

Parakeratosis

Polymorph microabscesses

Marked epidermal acanthosis

Dilated upper dermal capillaries

**Figure 8.1** Schematic representation of a psoriatic plaque.

This basic picture, with some variations (e.g. increased size and number of polymorph abscesses in pustular psoriasis), unites all forms of psoriasis and the skin lesions of Reiter's syndrome.

# Clinical patterns of psoriasis

A number of different clinical patterns are recognized. Some are common, others are rarer. We discuss them separately, but they may be seen together or overlap.

---

### Clinical patterns of psoriasis

- Classic plaque
- Scalp psoriasis
- Nail psoriasis
- Guttate
- Flexural
- 'Brittle'
- Erythrodermic
- Acute pustular
- Chronic palmoplantar pustulosis
- Arthropathic psoriasis

## Classic plaque psoriasis

This is the pattern that you will encounter most commonly. There are single or multiple red plaques, varying from a few millimetres to several centimetres in diameter, with a scaly surface (Figure 8.2). If scraped very gently, the scale can be seen to reflect the light, giving a 'silvery' effect (due to the parakeratotic horny layer). More vigorous rubbing induces capillary-point haemorrhage (Auspitz's sign).

The plaques may develop on any part of the body, but psoriasis has a predilection for extensor surfaces: the knees, the elbows and the base of the spine. Lesions are often strikingly symmetrical. Involvement of the face is relatively uncommon, but the scalp and nails are often affected (Figures 8.3 and 8.4), and an arthropathy may also occur.

Plaques tend to be chronic and stable, with little day-to-day change (compared with 'brittle' psoriasis—see below). However, they may enlarge slowly, merge with adjacent areas and also resolve spontaneously. Occasionally, psoriatic plaques appear at the site of trauma or scarring. This is known as the Koebner or isomorphic phenomenon and is a characteristic, but not pathognomonic, feature. Exposure to ultraviolet (UV) radiation and natural sunlight often (but not always) improves psoriasis.

Figure 8.2 Psoriatic plaque on the elbow.

Figure 8.3 Scalp psoriasis.

Figure 8.4 Nail pits in psoriasis.

It is often said that psoriasis is not itchy, but in our experience a significant number of patients complain of severe itching, and most experience some itch at times. In fact, the Greek *psora* actually means itch. Some forms of psoriasis (e.g. guttate, flexural) are more prone to cause irritation.

## Scalp psoriasis

Scalp involvement is very common: indeed the scalp may be affected alone. It can be difficult to distinguish scalp psoriasis from severe seborrhoeic dermatitis (see also Flexural psoriasis), but psoriasis lesions are generally thicker. As a rule of thumb, if you can feel scalp lesions as well as see them, they are probably psoriasis.

Involvement varies from one or two plaques to a sheet of thick scale covering the whole scalp surface (see Figure 8.3). Rarely, the scale becomes

Figure 8.5 Psoriatic onycholysis.

Figure 8.6 Guttate psoriasis.

very thick and sticks in large chunks to bundles of hair, a phenomenon known as 'pityriasis amiantacea'. There may be temporary hair loss in severe scalp psoriasis.

## Nail psoriasis

Nail abnormalities are frequent and are important diagnostic clues if skin lesions are few, or atypical. Nail changes are almost always present in arthropathic psoriasis.

Two common findings may occur together or alone: pitting and onycholysis. Psoriatic nail pits are relatively large and irregularly arranged (see Figure 8.4), compared with those of alopecia areata. Onycholysis (lifting of the nail plate) starts as a red–brown area and progresses to separation of the nail plate from the nail bed (Figure 8.5). It is sometimes painful. These nail changes, particularly onycholysis, may also occur without other evidence of the disease.

Occasionally, pustular changes occur at the ends of the digits and in the nail bed (sometimes known as 'acrodermatitis continua'). Similar changes may accompany chronic palmoplantar pustulosis (see below). In erythrodermic or pustular forms of psoriasis, the whole nail may become roughened and discoloured.

## Guttate psoriasis

Guttate psoriasis often develops suddenly, and may follow an infection, especially a streptococcal sore throat. It is a common way for psoriasis to present, particularly in young adults.

*Gutta* is the Latin for 'drop'. Most lesions are about a centimetre in diameter (Figure 8.6), and usually paler in colour than established plaque psoriasis, at least initially. The main differential diagnosis is pityriasis rosea (see Chapter 15), best distinguished by the presence of parakeratotic scale in psoriasis, and the shape of the lesions (round in guttate psoriasis, oval in pityriasis rosea). Guttate psoriasis may itch.

The lesions of guttate psoriasis often resolve rapidly, but in some patients the patches enlarge and become stable plaques.

## Flexural psoriasis

Flexural involvement in psoriasis may accompany typical plaque lesions, but is also commonly seen alone, or associated with scalp and nail changes. Lesions may occur in the groin, natal cleft, axillae, submammary folds and, importantly, umbilicus. Maceration inevitably occurs, and surface scale is often lost, leaving a rather beefy erythematous appearance (Figure 8.7). It may be difficult to

Figure 8.7 Flexural psoriasis.

distinguish this from flexural seborrhoeic dermatitis, so look for nail changes or evidence of psoriasis elsewhere. Some dermatologists believe in an overlap state between the two, and call such changes 'sebopsoriasis'.

Flexural psoriasis is often itchy. Watch out for a secondary contact sensitivity from the use of proprietary anti-itch preparations.

## Brittle psoriasis

Occasionally you will see patients whose psoriasis does not consist of thick, stable plaques, but of thin, irritable scaly areas (Figure 8.8). Lesions may arise anew or develop suddenly in a patient whose psoriasis has been stable for years. One reason for this is systemic steroid therapy (often for another condition), and potent topical steroids can also induce stable psoriasis to become 'brittle'.

The significance of brittle psoriasis is that the lesions are highly unstable and may rapidly generalize, especially if treated with potent agents (see Treatment below), leading to erythroderma (see Chapter 15) or even acute pustular psoriasis (see below).

## Erythrodermic psoriasis

When psoriatic plaques merge to involve most or all of the skin, a state of erythroderma or exfoliative dermatitis results. The effects of this are discussed in Chapter 15.

Psoriasis may become erythrodermic by slow inexorable progression, or very rapidly. Occasionally, new erythrodermic psoriasis may appear, and

Figure 8.8 Widespread 'brittle' psoriasis.

Figure 8.9 Acute pustular psoriasis.

(a)

may be precipitated by systemic steroids or potent topical steroids.

## Acute pustular psoriasis (of von Zumbusch)

This is a very serious condition. Patients with or without pre-existing psoriasis suddenly develop widespread erythema, superimposed on which are pustules. These may coalesce into lakes of pus (Figure 8.9). The pustules are sterile.

The patient has a high, swinging fever and is toxic and unwell, with a leukocytosis. If the disease is unchecked, patients become increasingly ill and may die, often of secondary infections.

## Chronic palmoplantar pustulosis (pustular psoriasis of palms and soles)

There is some debate about the relationship between this condition and other forms of psoriasis. Biopsies reveal psoriasiform pathology, but it is unusual for patients to have chronic palmoplantar pustulosis with other types of psoriasis.

The typical changes consist of erythematous patches with numerous pustules (Figure 8.10).

(b)

Figure 8.10 (a) Chronic palmoplantar pustulosis; (b) the sterile pustules dry to form circumscribed brown areas that are later shed.

These gradually change into brown, scaly spots and peel off. The condition is usually uncomfortable or painful, rather than itchy.

Lesions may involve only a small area of one hand or foot, or cover the entire surface of both palms and soles, leading to considerable disability.

# Treatment of psoriasis

The agents most widely used in the treatment of the skin lesions of psoriasis are given in the box.

---

**Agents for treating psoriasis**

**Topical**
- Emollients
- Tar
- Salicylic acid
- Topical steroids
- Dithranol (anthralin)
- Vitamin D analogues (e.g. calcipotriol, tacalcitol)
- Tazarotene
- Ultraviolet radiation

**Systemic**
- PUVA (psoralen + UVA)
- Retinoids
- Cytotoxics, e.g. methotrexate, azathioprine, hydroxycarbamide (hydroxyurea)
- Systemic steroids
- Ciclosporin
- 'Biologicals': various monoclonal antibodies

---

It is an old adage that if there are many treatments for a disease, none works perfectly; this is certainly true of psoriasis. Although each modality is useful in some patients, all represent a compromise in terms of safety, effectiveness and convenience. Many patients require a regimen of different agents for different sites at different times.

## Topical therapies

Many agents can be used topically to induce a remission or an improvement. Most are safe, but they are tedious for patients to use, as treatment may have to continue for months or, often, indefinitely.

## Emollients

Some patients are prepared to tolerate plaques (especially on covered sites) if scaling and discomfort can be controlled. Emollients such as white or yellow soft paraffin or lanolin may accomplish this.

## Salicylic acid

Salicylic acid is a 'keratolytic' agent and helps to reduce scaling. It can be used with tar in mixtures, and is also combined with a potent topical steroid in commercially available preparations.

## Tar

Tar has been used for many years, particularly in combination with UV radiation. The most effective preparations are extracts of crude coal tar. Attempts have been made to refine tar to make it more cosmetically acceptable, but the most effective forms still seem to be the darkest, smelliest and messiest. Consequently, not many patients will accept tar for widespread routine use. However, in bath oils or in ointment mixtures, tar may be helpful, and it is very valuable in scalp disease.

## Topical steroids

Topical steroids do not eradicate psoriasis, but may suppress it. Some dermatologists say that they never use topical steroids in psoriasis because of the risks (they may induce 'brittle' psoriasis). However, if used with care in stable disease, and on the scalp and in the flexures, they are undoubtedly useful.

## Dithranol (anthralin)

Dithranol is a curious substance that can convert psoriatic plaques into completely normal-looking skin. The mode of action is unknown. The 'Ingram regimen'—a combination of dithranol, tar and UV radiation—has been used for years: most patients can be cleared in about 3 weeks of daily treatment. Originally, dithranol was left on the skin for 24 h, but 'short-contact' therapy has been shown to be as good.

Dithranol works best in Lassar's paste (starch, zinc oxide and salicylic acid in white soft paraffin), but is also available in cream and ointment bases. Always begin with a low concentration (0.1%) and increase as necessary.

The main complications are staining (due to oxidation to a dye) and burning. Skin staining is temporary, but baths, bedding and clothes may be permanently marked. Dithranol burns can be very unpleasant, especially around the eyes and flexural areas. Patients must be taught to use dithranol carefully.

## Vitamin D analogues and tazarotene

Vitamin D analogues (calcipotriol, tacalcitol, calcitriol) work well, and have rapidly found a place in routine management. They may irritate the face and in the flexures, and calcium levels may be disturbed if large quantities of vitamin D analogues are applied. Tazarotene is a retinoid; patients using it should avoid pregnancy because of theoretical teratogenicity.

## Ultraviolet radiation

The use of UV therapy is well established, the most effective wavelengths being in the medium (UVB) range—and particularly 'narrow-band' UVB. UVB must be used with care because it also induces sunburn. Patients require doses that *just* induce erythema but do not cause burning. The dose is then increased gradually. Treatment is usually given two or three times weekly until clearance is achieved. Adjunctive tar may make UVB more effective.

UVB is theoretically carcinogenic (as is tar), but surprisingly few psoriasis sufferers develop skin cancers.

## Systemic therapies

### Psoralen + ultraviolet A (PUVA)

Psoralens form chemical bonds with DNA in the presence of UV radiation. The patient is given one of these agents (8-methoxypsoralen and trioxsalen are the most common), either as a soak or by mouth 2 h before exposure to long-wavelength UV light (UVA), initially twice weekly. Protective glasses are worn to prevent ocular damage. There is a significant long-term risk of keratoses and epithelial cancers with PUVA.

### Cytotoxic drugs

The most effective and widely used cytotoxic is methotrexate, a folic acid antagonist. Most psoriasis responds to a once-weekly dose of 7.5–20 mg. Other drugs occasionally used include azathioprine and hydroxycarbamide.

All cytotoxics have unwanted effects, particularly bone marrow suppression. This is rare with methotrexate, but may occur idiosyncratically, unrelated to dose. The major problem with methotrexate is hepatotoxicity, particularly fibrosis,

with chronic use. Alcohol appears to exacerbate this tendency. Patients require regular and continuous monitoring of liver function; it is now considered best practice to measure levels of a circulating collagen precursor (PIIINP). Sustained elevation indicates the need for a liver biopsy. Methotrexate also inhibits spermatogenesis and is teratogenic. Its use should therefore be restricted to severely affected patients.

## Retinoids

Vitamin A derivatives help some patients with psoriasis. The most commonly used is acitretin. Retinoids have a number of side effects, including dry lips, nose bleeds, hair loss, hyperlipidaemia, liver function test abnormalities and teratogenicity.

## Systemic steroids

In very severe psoriasis, especially erythrodermic or acute pustular forms, steroids may occasionally be necessary, but should not be used alone or for long.

## Ciclosporin

This immunosuppressive drug works extremely well, even in very severe psoriasis. It is nephrotoxic and very expensive.

## Biologicals (monoclonal antibodies)

A number of agents have been developed, aimed at specific compounds, e.g. TNF-$\alpha$, involved in immuno-inflammatory diseases such as rheumatoid arthritis and psoriasis. Examples include infliximab, etanercept and adalimumab. These are expensive, and can be used only under strict criteria in the UK. They all require administration by injection.

# Treatment of clinical patterns of psoriasis

The choice of therapeutic regimen in psoriasis is dictated by the type and extent of lesions, and by the effects on the patient's quality of life. A balance will often have to be struck between the need for improvement and the inconvenience and/or side effects of the agent(s) concerned.

## Chronic plaque psoriasis

Dithranol is a theoretical first choice, but patients' lifestyles, and treatment side effects often make it impractical. If so, vitamin D analogues or topical steroids (with or without tar and salicylic acid) are used. UV radiation may help. If lesions become very extensive, and/or if there are serious psychosocial problems, PUVA or systemic therapy may be indicated.

## Scalp psoriasis

Tar shampoos are helpful, but seldom control thick plaques alone. Tar gels may help, but the best topical remedy is Unguentum Cocois Co—a mixture including tar and salicylic acid. This is massaged in at night and washed out the following morning. Topical steroid lotions, with or without salicylic acid, are also useful.

## Nail psoriasis

Nail changes do not respond to topical treatment, and systemic drugs are seldom justified for nails alone.

## Guttate psoriasis

This is most effectively treated with UV radiation together with emollients and a tar-based ointment. If patients cannot find time to attend for treatment, a combination of moderately potent topical steroids and vitamin D analogues may be the best option.

## Flexural psoriasis

Psoriasis in the flexures poses problems. Mild tar/corticosteroid mixtures may be effective, but long-term use of topical steroids can cause striae. Dithranol, used in very low concentrations, can be successful, but burning is common and underclothes are stained. UVB and PUVA generally fail to reach the affected areas. Vitamin D analogues help, but can burn. Tacrolimus and pimecrolimus have been used recently (and for facial lesions).

## Brittle psoriasis

Brittle psoriasis requires careful management. Avoid potent topical steroids, strong tar and salicylic acid preparations. Emollients or very dilute steroids may bring the skin into a more stable condition, but PUVA, retinoids or methotrexate may be needed, at least for a short time.

## Erythrodermic and acute pustular psoriasis

Although both of these states may settle with conservative management, it is more likely that systemic treatment will be required. Such intervention can be life saving. The most common choice is methotrexate, but ciclosporin also works well. Once the condition has stabilized, the dose should be gradually reduced and the drug stopped if possible. However, many patients relapse and require long-term treatment. Biologicals may become an important option in such patients.

## Chronic palmoplantar pustulosis

Nothing really works well in this condition. Tar pastes, potent topical steroids or dithranol are often ineffective. Vitamin D analogues may be worth a trial, as is oral acitretin, and PUVA to the hands and feet may provide control, but relapse is common with any therapy.

# Arthropathic psoriasis

One of the most unpleasant complications of psoriasis is arthropathy, affecting up to 10% of people with psoriasis. There are four basic patterns as shown in the box.

---

**Psoriatic arthropathy patterns**

- Distal interphalangeal joint involvement
- Seronegative rheumatoid-like joint changes
- Large joint mono- or polyarthropathy
- Spondylitis

---

Most commonly the distal interphalangeal joints are involved, with the other changes listed in the box in descending order of frequency. Psoriatic arthropathy is erosive and may result in joint destruction if left unchecked.

People with psoriasis who develop spondylitis are usually HLA-B27 positive, and there is overlap between psoriatic arthropathy and other seronegative arthritides.

Non-steroidal anti-inflammatory drugs and methotrexate are used. Biologicals are gaining particular importance in this group of patients.

## Reiter's syndrome

This disorder, which frequently follows a diarrhoeal illness or non-specific urethritis in HLA-B27-positive individuals, is discussed in Chapter 19. Occasionally skin lesions known as 'keratoderma blennorrhagicum' develop. Palmar and plantar lesions may become gross (Figure 8.11), and lesions elsewhere are clinically very similar to psoriasis. Histologically, they are indistinguishable.

Figure 8.11 Keratoderma blennorrhagicum.

# 9

# Benign and malignant skin tumours

*Lecture Notes: Dermatology*, 10th edition. © RAC Graham-Brown and DA Burns. Published 2011 by Blackwell Publishing Ltd.

*Know ye not that a little leaven leaveneth the whole lump?*

*St Paul (1 Corinthians, 5:6)*

## Introduction: classification of skin tumours

Lumps on or in the skin are extremely common and the workload associated with them is rising because of the following:

1 The age of the population is increasing (many skin tumours are more common in elderly people)
2 The incidence of skin cancer is increasing in all age groups
3 There is increasing public awareness of skin tumours and their potential importance

Most skin tumours are benign, often representing only a cosmetic nuisance. However, it is important to distinguish these from malignant or potentially malignant tumours quickly and effectively, as practical decisions about a lesion can be made only after a diagnosis to this minimum level.

Benign and malignant tumours are described for every component of the skin. Table 9.1 presents a simplified version of the wide variety that may be encountered.

## General treatment principles for skin tumours

It is worth reviewing briefly the techniques used to treat skin tumours to avoid repetition.

The first important principle is that, unless the diagnosis is certain, some tissue should always be preserved for histology. Failure to do this will mean missed malignancies, and is one explanation for patients who present with mysterious lymphatic or distant deposits from unknown primary sites.

### Surgical removal or biopsy

These techniques have already been described and illustrated (Figures 2.2–2.4). Removal of small skin tumours is quick, simple and economical. If the tumour is too large for primary excision, a small incisional biopsy, crossing the edge from normal to abnormal tissue, should be taken. There is no evidence that such a biopsy adversely affects the outcome, although it is advisable to avoid incisional biopsy of suspected invasive melanomas if possible (see below).

### Curettage and/or cautery ('C&C')

This is a perfectly satisfactory method for the removal of superficial tumours.

**Table 9.1 Tumours, benign or malignant, found in the epidermis and dermis**

| Types of tumours | Types of tumours |
|---|---|
| A Epidermis (for naevi see Chapter 10) | C: Dermis (for naevi see Chapter 10) |
| *Benign* | *Benign* |
| • Seborrhoeic keratosis | • Fibrous tissue: |
| • Skin tags | — dermatofibroma |
| • Keratoacanthoma | • 'Neural' tissue, e.g. neurofibroma |
| • Viral warts (see Chapter 3) | • Vascular tissue: |
| • Clear cell acanthoma | — angioma/angiokeratoma |
| • Tumours of skin appendages, e.g. sweat glands, sebaceous glands, hair follicles | — pyogenic granuloma |
| • Epidermal cysts | — glomus tumour |
| *Dysplastic/malignant* | *Dysplastic/malignant* |
| • Basal cell carcinoma | • Fibrosarcoma |
| • Actinic (solar) keratosis | • Neurofibrosarcoma |
| • Squamous cell carcinoma: | • Angiosarcoma, including Kaposi's sarcoma |
| — *in situ* (Bowen's disease) | D Pseudo-tumours |
| — invasive | • Chondrodermatitis nodularis helicis |
| • Paget's disease | • Hypertrophic and keloid scars |
| • Tumours of skin appendages | E Lymphomas |
| B Melanocytes (for naevi see Chapter 10) | • Cutaneous T-cell lymphoma (mycosis fungoides) |
| *Benign* | • Cutaneous B-cell lymphoma |
| • Freckle and lentigo | F Extension from deeper tissues |
| *Dysplastic/malignant* | G Metastatic deposits |
| • Dysplastic naevus (see Chapter 10) | |
| • Lentigo maligna | |
| • Malignant melanoma: | |
| — lentigo maligna melanoma | |
| — superficial spreading | |
| — nodular | |
| — acral | |

**C&C**

1 Anaesthetise the area
2 Use a curette (Volkmann spoon) to scrape off lesions
3 Touch the raw base a few times with cautery or a hyfrecator* to control oozing
4 Apply a simple dressing and/or antiseptic

*A hyfrecator produces electrical haemostasis and desiccation.

Pedunculated tumours can be removed by slicing with cautery across the base.

## Cryotherapy

The use of cryotherapy for tumours has become very popular. It is ideal for superficial skin tumours because it is quick and leaves relatively little scarring. However, histological interpretation of cryobiopsies is not easy and it should be used only if the tumour is considered to be definitely benign. Cryotherapy is not appropriate for melanomas. The best agent is liquid nitrogen.

## Cryotherapy

1 Apply nitrogen with cotton-wool buds, or by specially designed spray or probe instruments

2 Wait until a halo of frozen skin 1 mm around the tumour is obtained

3 Maintain halo for 10 s for benign, 30 s for malignant tumours

4 Allow to thaw, and repeat (two 'freeze/thaw cycles')

The patient should be told to expect blistering, followed by healing with crust formation. The lesion should separate within 3 weeks.

## Radiotherapy

Radiotherapy is an effective treatment method for basal (BCC) and squamous cell carcinomas (SCC), and may be the most practical option for very large tumours in elderly patients. However, it is not ideal for trunk and limb lesions.

Radiotherapy can also control secondary tumour deposits.

## Lasers and photodynamic therapy

There is an increasing interest in the application of laser technology to treating skin disease, especially for skin tumours and naevi (see Chapter 10), but also for hirsutism (see Chapter 13), scars, wrinkles and other 'defects'. Many benign epithelial tumours will respond to ablation by a $CO_2$ laser but are also very easily treated by other, simpler, cheaper means. Pigmented lesions respond to lasers, but their place has yet to be fully established.

Photodynamic therapy (PDT) is a process involving the application of a porphyrin and exposure to light. It is useful for widespread superficial lesions such as Bowen's disease and superficial BCC.

# Specific tumours

We first consider benign tumours, and then dysplastic and malignant processes, discussing the most common and most important of these.

Some skin lumps are hamartomatous malformations. Such a lesion in the skin is termed a 'naevus'. Naevi are discussed separately in Chapter 10.

## Benign tumours—epidermal

## Seborrhoeic keratoses (seborrhoeic warts, basal cell papillomas)

You are bound to see seborrhoeic keratoses, if only in passing while examining a chest. They are most frequent in elderly people, and may be solitary or multiple. Occasionally there are hundreds (a tendency that may be familial).

### Clinical features

A flat-topped area of skin with a 'stuck-on' appearance (Figure 9.1). They may be pale, but are often

Figure 9.1 Typical seborrhoeic warts.

pigmented, sometimes deeply so. The surface is often said to be greasy, but a more useful sign is the granular look occasioned by small surface pits and irregularities.

### Sites of predilection

Head and neck; backs of hands and forearms; trunk.

### Differential diagnosis

Usually straightforward, but darkly pigmented lesions can be mistaken for melanomas. On the face, seborrhoeic keratoses may remain virtually flat, causing difficulty in distinguishing them from senile lentigo or lentigo maligna (see below). Another diagnostic problem arises if lesions become inflamed. There may be crusting and bleeding, and biopsy for histology may be necessary.

### Treatment

If deemed necessary (there is no malignant potential), the best approach for smaller lesions is cryotherapy. Larger ones may be better treated by C & C or excision.

## Skin tags (acrochordons)

Many people develop these small pedunculated lesions around the neck and in the axillae. Increasing age and obesity are predisposing factors.

### Differential diagnosis

Small melanocytic naevi may look similar, and so may small pedunculated seborrhoeic keratoses.

### Treatment

They can be removed very easily by snip and cautery/hyfrecation.

## Keratoacanthoma

This tumour is an oddity. Some authors classify keratoacanthoma as malignant because the histology so closely resembles that of SCC (see below). Keratoacanthomas are much more common on sun-exposed skin and in elderly people.

### Clinical features

Lesions arise rapidly, reaching a maximal size over the course of 6–8 weeks (see Figure 9.2). Tumours are round, with rolled edges and a

Figure 9.2 Keratoacanthoma.

central keratin plug. The base is often red and inflamed, and may be painful. Ultimately, the lesion begins to shrink, often almost as quickly as it enlarged, and disappears completely, leaving a small puckered scar.

### Sites of predilection

Head and neck, forearms and hands.

### Differential diagnosis

Differentiation from BCC (see below) can be made on the basis of the history of rapid growth and the remarkable round architecture.

The challenge is to distinguish *prospectively* between a keratoacanthoma and a SCC. By definition a keratoacanthoma should resolve spontaneously, but this cannot be determined in advance. Incisional biopsies may not help because of the close similarities to SCC.

## Treatment

It is reasonable to wait expectantly for a short while if a lesion is very typical, especially in a frail patient. However, if there is any diagnostic doubt, keratoacanthomas are best removed and sent for histology. There is a case for removing such a lesion early, to avoid a more complex procedure if it becomes much larger.

## Other benign epidermal tumours

Viral warts are discussed in Chapter 3, and the other benign epidermal tumours listed are rare.

## Epidermal cysts

There are three common forms of epidermal cyst—pilar, epidermoid (frequently, but quite wrongly, called 'sebaceous') and the milium.

1 Common scalp cysts are correctly termed 'pilar' or 'trichilemmal' cysts. There may be several, and a familial predisposition is usual
2 Epidermoid cysts may be found anywhere, but are most common on the head, neck and trunk. They often follow severe acne; there is a cystic swelling within the skin, usually with an overlying punctum. *Treatment*: both types can be removed easily under local anaesthetic using a linear incision over the surface
3 Milia are extremely common. They may occur spontaneously or after trauma or blistering. In some families, there is an inherited tendency to develop clusters on the cheeks and around the eyes (see Figure 9.3). *Treatment*: milia can be treated by incision, pricking out or cautery/ hyfrecation

## Benign melanocytic tumours

### Freckles (ephelides) and lentigines

Freckles are areas of skin containing melanocytes, normal in number but hyperresponsive to UV radiation. They are genetically determined: we all know typical freckly red heads.

Lentigines are flat pigmented areas composed of increased numbers of melanocytes.

Melanocytic naevi are discussed in Chapter 10.

## Benign tumours—dermal

### Dermatofibromas

Dermatofibromas (Figure 9.4) consist of a mixture of histiocytes, fibrous tissue and blood vessels. It is not known why they occur, but they may follow minor trauma.

### Clinical features

More common in women; often easier to diagnose by touch than by sight—they feel like small lentils.

### Sites of predilection

Limbs; legs more than arms.

Figure 9.3 Milia around the eyes: a characteristic site.

Figure 9.4 Dermatofibroma (histiocytoma).

## Differential diagnosis

Occasionally, heavy pigmentation can cause confusion with melanoma.

## Treatment

Excision may be cosmetically indicated.

## Angiomas

Angiomas are collections of aberrant blood vessels within the dermis and/or subcutaneous tissues. Some are developmental defects, commonly present at birth, and these are discussed in Chapter 10. Others develop during adult life, such as the ubiquitous Campbell de Morgan spot (Figure 9.5).

## Pyogenic granulomas

Pyogenic granulomas are benign reactive inflammatory masses composed of blood vessels and fibroblasts.

### Clinical features

They erupt rapidly, usually have a polypoid appearance (Figure 9.6) and a 'collar' around the base; profuse contact bleeding is common.

### Sites of predilection

Sites of an injury or infection, often on a digit.

### Differential diagnosis

They must be differentiated from SCCs and amelanotic melanomas.

### Treatment

Removal by curettage or excision should always be followed by histological examination.

## Others

You may encounter several other benign dermal or subcutaneous lumps: e.g. neurofibromas in von

Figure 9.5 Campbell de Morgan spots.

Figure 9.6 Side view of a typical pyogenic granuloma.

Recklinghausen's neurofibromatosis (see Chapter 11); various benign fibroblastic tumours; and lipomas, which are readily identified by their soft texture and lobulated outline.

If there is any doubt about any dermal or subcutaneous lump, it is best removed for histology.

## Pseudo-tumours

### Chondrodermatitis nodularis helicis (painful nodule of the ear)

This curious lesion is not a tumour, but an inflammatory process.

#### Clinical features

A small umbilicated nodule on the rim of the ear, more commonly in men (Figure 9.7); the clue is that it is painful—often exquisitely so—especially in bed at night.

#### Differential diagnosis

It is often confused with BCCs or other tumours.

#### Treatment

Cryotherapy has become popular but we prefer excision, with paring down of adjacent cartilage.

### Hypertrophic scars and keloids

Scar formation can be very exuberant, especially at some sites (see below) and in children, young

Figure 9.7 Chondrodermatitis nodularis helicis.

adults and black skin. A hypertrophic scar flattens after about 2 years, whereas a keloid persists and spreads laterally beyond the original site (keloids can become very large).

### Clinical features

Protuberant masses usually after cuts, ear piercing, burns, acne and BCG inoculations performed high on the shoulder; some appear to develop spontaneously; keloids often itch.

### Sites of predilection

Chest, upper back, shoulder, pubic region, ear lobes.

### Differential diagnosis

Any soft-tissue tumour, especially if there is no preceding history of trauma.

### Treatment

Management can be extremely difficult. Biopsy may be necessary if there is diagnostic doubt but any surgery, especially excision, generally leads to recurrence and can make matters worse. Intralesional steroids and the use of silica gels have their advocates.

## Dysplastic and malignant tumours

The term 'dysplasia' implies that the skin has been partly, or wholly, replaced by cells with neoplastic features. When this results in invasion of adjacent tissue, the process can genuinely be said to be 'malignant'.

Cutaneous dysplasias and malignancies are increasingly common, especially in ageing skin and in skin exposed to prolonged UV radiation. Other factors are also associated with dysplastic skin changes:

1 Most forms of ionizing radiation (UV, X-rays, γ-rays) are powerful inducers of skin cancer
2 There are several known carcinogens, notably industrial oils, tars and bitumen; exposure to soot caused scrotal cancers in chimney sweeps
3 Skin cancers are a feature of some genetic diseases: a notable example is xeroderma pigmentosum, in which repair of UV-induced DNA damage is faulty
4 Skin cancers are more common in immunosuppressed individuals, especially after renal and cardiac transplantation and in HIV/AIDS

## Dysplastic/malignant epidermal tumours

### Basal cell carcinoma

The most common malignant skin tumour, at least in white skin, is often known as a 'rodent ulcer'.

### Clinical features

Most begin as a nodule (Figure 9.8) which spreads slowly outwards, usually leaving a central depression (creating the classic 'rolled edge'); usually skin coloured with a translucent look (often described as 'pearly'); telangiectatic vessels on the

Figure 9.8 Basal cell carcinoma: note the telangiectatic vessels.

surface are very characteristic, and account for contact bleeding being a common symptom; metastasis is extremely rare, but local invasion can be destructive (Figure 9.9) and BCCs can spread along bony passages into the skull.

Figure 9.9 Basal cell carcinoma: such destruction gives rise to the term 'rodent ulcer'.

## Variants

Several distinctive clinical variants of the BCC are recognized (see below).

### Sites of predilection

Predominantly the face, but BCCs occur on other sun-exposed sites, in the hair-bearing scalp, behind the ear and on the trunk (where the superficial pattern is common).

### Differential diagnosis

Early lesions may be confused with naevi; superficial BCCs are often treated as inflammatory; heavy pigmentation may suggest a melanoma; morphoeic tumours can be very difficult to diagnose.

---

**Clinical variants of BCC**

- Nodular: nodule with central depression and a rolled edge; surface telangiectasia
- Morphoeic: a flat growth pattern which results in a scar-like appearance; it can be very difficult to know where the tumour begins and ends, and local invasion is more common
- Superficial: lesions grow for many years and may be many centimetres across; usually solitary; multiple tumours may indicate previous arsenic ingestion; characteristically, a 'worm-like' edge is seen (Figure 9.10)
- Pigmented: pigmentation is usually patchy but may be very dark and dense

---

Figure 9.10 Superficial basal cell carcinoma.

## Treatment

Excision, biopsy and radiotherapy or, for superficial tumours, curettage, cryotherapy or photodynamic therapy; careful assessment of morphoeic tumours is needed—a technique known as 'microscopically controlled surgery' (Mohs' surgery) may be helpful because it allows prospective delineation of tumour extent. It is particularly important to deal adequately with lesions around the eyes, nose and ears. The use of topical therapies for superficial types, notably imiquimod (a promoter of interferon-α), has been pioneered more recently.

## Actinic or solar keratoses

These are areas of dysplastic squamous epithelium without invasion, but actinic keratoses do have low-grade malignant potential and their presence indicates unstable epithelium.

### Clinical features

Red and scaly patches (Figure 9.11) that characteristically wax and wane with time; many hundreds of lesions may occur in heavily sun-exposed individuals.

### Sites of predilection

Light-exposed skin, especially the face, forearms, dorsa of hands, lower legs and bald scalp.

### Differential diagnosis

Lesions of chronic discoid lupus erythematosus can be difficult to distinguish, and some are pigmented, leading to confusion with lentigo maligna (see below).

### Treatment

Cryotherapy is best for small numbers of lesions; large areas on the face and scalp can be treated with the topical agents diclofenac sodium, 5-fluorouracil, imiquimod; in very elderly patients it may be best to do nothing.

## Squamous cell carcinoma *in situ* (or Bowen's disease)

Bowen's disease is an SCC confined to the epidermis, and is common below the knees in elderly women. Invasive change does occur but is rare.

Figure 9.11 Multiple solar keratoses.

### Clinical features

Usually a solitary patch of red scaly skin, although multiple areas may occur; Bowen's disease is asymptomatic.

### Variant

Erythroplasia of Queyrat—non-invasive dysplastic changes may also occur on the penis, where the clinical appearance is of a velvety red plaque. Although given a separate name, it is essentially the same as Bowen's disease elsewhere.

### Sites of predilection

Light-exposed skin; may occur on non-exposed areas such as the trunk.

### Differential diagnosis

There is a superficial resemblance to psoriasis (Figure 9.12), but the surface scale is adherent rather than flaky and removal of scale leaves a glistening red surface, not bleeding. Arsenic was

Figure 9.12 Two patches of Bowen's disease.

Figure 9.13 Paget's disease of the nipple.

once used to treat psoriasis, so keep an eye out for Bowen's disease in elderly individuals with psoriasis.

Similar changes on one nipple should always suggest the possibility of Paget's disease (Figure 9.13); a biopsy should be performed because there is always an underlying breast carcinoma.

## Treatment

Should be treated by excision, curettage, cryotherapy or photodynamic therapy; very large areas may require radiotherapy.

# Invasive squamous cell carcinomas

SCCs are locally invasive, and may metastasize to regional lymph nodes and beyond (especially lip, mouth and genital lesions). UV radiation is important aetiologically, but other factors also play a role: smoking in lip and mouth cancers; wart virus in genital lesions.

## Clinical features

These may be very varied, typically:

1 a keratotic lump
2 a rapidly growing polypoid mass (Figure 9.14)
3 a cutaneous ulcer

SCCs are often surrounded by actinic keratoses.

## Sites of predilection

Sun-exposed sites; SCCs also develop on the lips (Figure 9.15), in the mouth and on the genitalia.

Figure 9.14 A polypoid squamous cell carcinoma.

Figure 9.15 Squamous cell carcinoma on the lip.

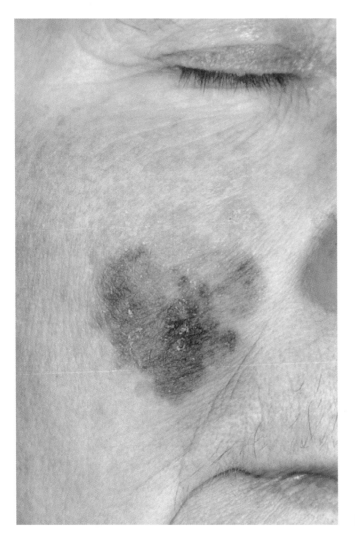

Figure 9.16 Lentigo maligna.

### Differential diagnosis

Keratotic lesions may closely resemble hypertrophic actinic keratoses.

### Treatment

Biopsy of any suspicious lesion; definitive treatment is by surgical removal or radiotherapy.

## Dysplastic/malignant melanocytic tumours

### Lentigo maligna (or Hutchinson's malignant freckle)

The term 'lentigo maligna' describes a patch of malignant melanocytes, in sun-damaged skin, which proliferate radially along the dermoepidermal junction and deep around hair follicles, often for many years. An invasive component may develop at any time.

### Clinical features

A flat brown area with irregular pigmentation.

### Sites of predilection

Almost always on the face (Figure 9.16).

### Differential diagnosis

Can be difficult to distinguish from flat seborrhoeic keratoses, pigmented actinic keratoses and simple lentigines.

### Treatment

Biopsy is essential; definitive treatment is a matter of debate; excision is our preferred option because of the risk of recurrences with cryotherapy or topical therapies; in very elderly patients it may be reasonable to do nothing and follow the patient carefully.

---

### Malignant melanoma patterns

**Lentigo maligna melanoma**
The appearance of a nodule of invasive melanoma within a lentigo maligna.

**Superficial spreading melanoma (SSM)**
The most common in the UK; the tumour has a radial growth phase before true invasion begins
- Clinical features:
  — irregularly pigmented brown/black patch with an irregular edge (Figure 9.17)
  — may itch or give rise to mild discomfort
  — may bleed
- Sites of predilection: most frequently on the leg in women and the trunk in men, but may occur anywhere
- Differential diagnosis:
  — naevi in the young
  — flat seborrhoeic keratoses in older patients

**Nodular melanoma**
The tumour exhibits an invasive growth pattern from the outset
- Clinical features:
  — rapidly growing lumps (Figure 9.18)
  — occasionally warty (verrucous melanoma) or non-pigmented (amelanotic melanoma)
- Sites of predilection: may occur anywhere
- Differential diagnosis: other rapidly growing tumours

**Acral melanoma**
Rare in the UK, but much more common in other countries (e.g. Japan); it is virtually the only type of melanoma seen in Asian or African–Caribbean patients
- Clinical feature: a pigmented patch on the sole or palm or an area of subungual pigmentation
- Differential diagnosis:
  — can be confused with a viral wart
  — must be distinguished from haematoma

Some malignant melanomas arise in pre-existing melanocytic naevi, although estimates of the frequency of this vary from 5% to over 50%

Figure 9.17 Superficial spreading melanoma.

Figure 9.18 Large nodular melanoma.

## Malignant melanoma

This is the most dangerous of the three most common malignant skin tumours. Melanomas, other than lentigo maligna melanoma, occur in a relatively younger age group than other skin cancers. The incidence continues to rise, even in temperate climates, probably as a result of the intermittent sun exposure that has become so fashionable. Rising standards of living have permitted more leisure time at home and abroad, during which the most important 'activity' is sunbathing.

Exposure to very strong sunlight with sunburn is particularly risky and childhood sun exposure may be important. Some melanomas arise in pre-existing melanocytic naevi (see Chapter 10). It seems that the incidence of this varies from country to country.

There are four recognized patterns of malignant melanoma (see box).

### Treatment of malignant melanoma

The prognosis in malignant melanoma is related to the depth of tumour invasion, regardless of the original type. It is standard practice to measure this using a technique known as the 'Breslow thickness' (Figure 9.19). In tumours <1.5 mm at first excision, 5-year survival rate is about 90%; if the depth is >3.5 mm this falls to 40% or less.

All types of melanoma should therefore be excised as soon as possible. Radiotherapy and chemotherapy have little to offer in curing the disease. There is some debate about how wide excision margins should be, but there is no harm in initial narrow excision. The urgency is to remove the melanoma—further procedures can be considered later.

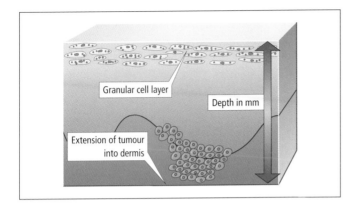

Figure 9.19 Breslow thickness.

In acral melanoma it may be necessary to perform a confirmatory biopsy before definitive treatment, which may involve amputation.

### Encouraging early presentation

The most effective way of improving treatment is to increase public awareness of malignant melanomas and thereby prompt people to seek advice about suspicious lesions. Many doctors now use a checklist (see box).

---

**Malignant melanoma checklist**

- Is an existing mole getting larger or a new one growing? After puberty, moles usually do not grow. (This sign essentially refers to adults, remember that naevi may grow rapidly in children (see Chapter 10).)
- Does the lesion have an irregular outline? Ordinary moles are a smooth, regular shape
- Is the lesion irregularly pigmented? Particularly, is there a mixture of shades of brown and black?
- Is the lesion larger than 1 cm in diameter?
- Is the lesion inflamed or is there a reddish edge?
- Is the lesion bleeding, oozing or crusting?
- Does the lesion itch or hurt?

Any pigmented lesion, whether newly arising or already present, that exhibits three or more of the seven listed features, and especially one of the first three, should be treated as highly suspicious.

---

## Prevention of epithelial and melanocytic malignancies

Both types of epithelial skin cancer, and melanoma, are more common in those who burn easily in the sun: those with fair skin, fair or red hair, and blue or green eyes (skin types I and II—see Chapter 12). Melanomas are also more common in individuals with many melanocytic naevi.

It is logical therefore to recommend that those at risk avoid excessive sun exposure:

1 No one should allow him- or herself to be sunburnt
2 It is best to avoid midday sun or, at least, wear adequate clothing and hats
3 Sun-screens offering a high degree of protection should be used

Those who tan easily and those with brown or black skin need not take such draconian precautions, but for all children sun exposure should be restricted.

## Dermal malignant tumours

Malignant sarcomas may develop in the skin.

### Clinical features

Indolent, slow-growing nodules, which become fixed to deeper tissues.

### Differential diagnosis

Difficult to categorize without biopsy.

### Treatment

Wide excision; in one tumour of this kind (dermatofibrosarcoma protuberans), very wide indeed.

## Kaposi's sarcoma

This malignant vascular tumour merits special mention in spite of its rarity. 'Classic' Kaposi's sarcoma occurs in Ashkenazi Jews and northern Italians. A much more aggressive form is seen in Africans and in people with HIV/AIDS.

### Clinical features

Purplish plaques and nodules.

### Sites of predilection

Legs in the classic form; anywhere in the aggressive form.

### Differential diagnosis

Other vascular lesions.

### Treatment

Biopsy; treatment of underlying condition; symptomatic treatment with radiotherapy may help occasionally.

## Lymphomas

Lymphomatous involvement of the skin may be secondary, e.g. in non-Hodgkin's B-cell lymphoma. However, the skin may be the original site, especially in cutaneous T-cell lymphoma (often called 'mycosis fungoides').

### Clinical features

Variable; some areas remain unchanged or grow slowly for years; red, well-circumscribed, scaly plaques, tumours and ulceration eventually develop (Figure 9.20).

### Differential diagnosis

Lesions can be confused with eczema or psoriasis.

### Treatment

Biopsy is essential but can be difficult to interpret. DNA phenotyping of cells may be of value; defini-

**Figure 9.20** Areas of mycosis fungoides (cutaneous T-cell lymphoma).

tive treatment varies with the stage, but includes radiotherapy, PUVA, interferon-α and various chemotherapeutic regimens.

# Extension from deeper tissues and metastases

Tumours of underlying structures, such as breast, may invade the skin. The skin may also be the site of metastatic deposits from internal cancers such as bronchogenic carcinoma (see Chapter 19).

# 10

# Naevi

*Ten thousand saw I at a glance*
*William Wordsworth, 'The Daffodils'*

## Introduction

Naevi are extremely common—virtually everyone has some. We use the word 'naevus' to mean a cutaneous hamartoma (a lesion in which normal tissue components are present in abnormal quantities or patterns). This encompasses 'naevi' that are not actually present at birth, because the cells from which they arise are. The word can give rise to confusion, largely because it is used by some writers more loosely, e.g. the word for melanocytic naevi may not strictly be applied without further qualification (see below). This is complicated further by some 'naevi' being called 'moles' or 'birthmarks'. Thus, a lump described as a 'mole' may be a melanocytic naevus, but may also be any small skin lesion, especially if pigmented, whereas 'birthmark' is accurate enough as far as it goes, but many naevi develop after birth.

Any component of the skin may produce a naevus, and they may be classified accordingly (Table 10.1). We need discuss only the most important: epithelial and organoid naevi, vascular naevi and melanocytic naevi.

## Epithelial and 'organoid' naevi

These are relatively uncommon developmental defects of epidermal structures: the epidermis

*Lecture Notes: Dermatology*, 10th edition. © RAC Graham-Brown and DA Burns. Published 2011 by Blackwell Publishing Ltd.

itself, hair follicles and sebaceous glands. There are two important types: the epidermal naevus and the sebaceous naevus.

### Epidermal naevus

Circumscribed areas of epidermal thickening may be present at birth or develop during childhood; many are linear. Very rarely, there are associated central nervous system (CNS) abnormalities.

Becker's naevus presents as a pigmented patch first seen at or around puberty, usually on the upper trunk or shoulder, and which gradually enlarges and frequently also becomes increasingly hairy.

### Sebaceous naevus

Sebaceous naevi are easily overlooked at birth. They begin as flat, yellow areas on the head and neck which, in the hairy scalp, may cause localized alopecia. Later, the naevus becomes thickened and warty, and basal cell carcinomas may arise within it. These naevi are best excised during adolescence.

## Melanocytic naevi

The most common naevi are formed from melanocytes that have failed to mature or migrate properly during embryonic development. We all have some. Look at your own skin or, better, that of an attractive classmate, to see typical examples!

It is convenient to categorize melanocytic naevi by clinical and histopathological features, because there are relevant differences (see Table 10.1). The first is whether they are present at birth (congenital) or arise later (acquired).

### Table 10.1 A classification of naevi

**Epithelial and 'organoid'**
- Epidermal naevus
- Sebaceous naevus

**Melanocytic**

*Congenital*
- Congenital melanocytic naevus
- Mongolian blue spot

*Acquired*
- Junctional/compound/intradermal naevus
- Sutton's halo naevus
- Dysplastic naevus
- Blue naevus
- Spitz naevus

**Vascular**

*Telangiectatic*
- Superficial capillary naevus
- Deep capillary naevus
- Rare telangiectatic disorders

*Angiomatous*

**Other tissues**
- Connective tissue
- Mast cell
- Fat

Figure 10.1 Giant congenital melanocytic naevus.

## Congenital

### Congenital melanocytic naevus

It is widely reported that 1% of children have a melanocytic naevus at birth.

These vary from a few millimetres to many centimetres in diameter. There is a rare, but huge and grossly disfiguring variant, the 'giant' congenital melanocytic or 'bathing trunk' naevus (Figure 10.1).

Small-to-medium congenital melanocytic naevi may be very slightly more prone to develop melanomas than acquired lesions, but the giant type presents a high risk, even early in childhood. Prepubertal malignant melanoma is extremely rare, but nearly always involves a congenital naevus. The therapeutic paradox is that small, low-risk lesions are easily removed but surgery for larger lesions with unquestioned malignant potential is simply impractical. Each case must be judged on its own merits. Decisions must involve the parents/carers and the child.

### Mongolian blue spot

Most children of Mongoloid extraction and many south Asian and African–Caribbean babies are born with a diffuse blue–black patch on the lower back and buttocks. There are melanocytes widely dispersed in the dermis (the depth is responsible for the colour). The area fades as the child grows, but may persist indefinitely. Unwary doctors have mistaken Mongolian blue spots for bruising, and accused parents of baby battering.

## Acquired

### Acquired melanocytic naevus

A melanocytic naevus is 'acquired' if it develops during postnatal life, a phenomenon that is so common as to be 'normal'. Most only represent a

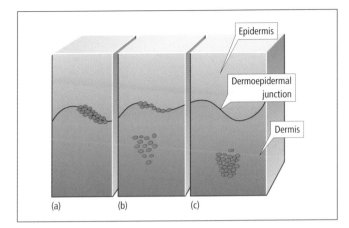

Figure 10.2 The phases of the acquired melanocytic naevus: (a) junctional; (b) compound; (c) intradermal. These stages are part of a continuum, and each lasts a variable time.

minor nuisance, and 'beauty spots' were once highly fashionable.

The first thing to understand is that each naevus has its own life history. This will make the terms applied to the different stages in their evolution clearer (Figure 10.2).

The lesion (Figure 10.3) is first noticed when immature melanocytes proliferate at the dermoepidermal junction (hence 'junctional'). After a variable period of radial growth, some cells drop into the dermis ('compound'). Eventually the junctional element disappears and all melanocytic cells are within the dermis ('intradermal'). Different melanocytic naevi will be at different stages of development in the same individual.

Most melanocytic naevi appear in the first 20 years of life, but may continue to develop well into the 40s. They are initially pigmented, often heavily and even alarmingly, but later may become pale, especially when intradermal. Most disappear altogether: very few octogenarians have many.

Their importance (apart from cosmetic) is threefold:

1 Some malignant melanomas develop in a pre-existing naevus (the chance of this happening in any one lesion, though, is infinitesimally small)
2 The possession of large numbers of acquired melanocytic naevi is statistically associated with an increased risk of melanoma
3 Melanocytic naevi can be confused with melanomas

Any melanocytic lesion that behaves oddly should be excised and sent for histology. Remember, however, that by definition all melanocytic naevi grow at some stage. Therefore, growth alone is not necessarily sinister, especially in younger individuals. Most naevi undergoing malignant change show features outlined in Chapter 9, but 'if in doubt, lop it out'!

There are several variants of the acquired melanocytic naevus (see box).

---

**Acquired melanocytic naevus**

Sutton's halo naevus: a white ring develops around an otherwise typical melanocytic naevus; the lesion may become paler and disappear (Figure 10.4). This is an immune response of no sinister significance and unknown cause

Dysplastic naevus: some lesions look unusual and/or have unusual histopathological features; this may affect just one or two naevi, but some people have many; such individuals may be part of a pedigree in which there is a striking increase in melanoma ('dysplastic naevus syndrome')

Blue naevus: the characteristic slate-blue colour (Figure 10.5) is due to clusters of melanocytes lying deep in the dermis; they are most common on the extremities, head and buttocks

Spitz naevus: these lesions have a characteristic brick-red colour; Spitz naevi have occasionally been confused histologically with malignant melanoma

Figure 10.3 The development phases of an acquired melanocytic naevus: (a) junctional (flat, pigmented); (b) compound (raised, pigmented); (c) intradermal (raised, no pigment).

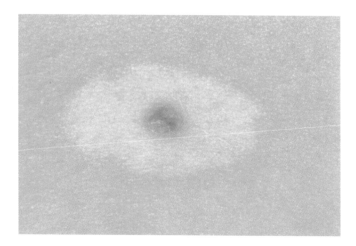

Figure 10.4 Sutton's 'halo' naevus.

Figure 10.5 Blue naevus.

Figure 10.6 Superficial capillary naevus.

# Vascular naevi

Vascular blemishes are common. Some present relatively minor problems, whereas others are very disfiguring. The terminology used for these lesions can be confusing and is by no means uniform. We have adopted what we consider to be a simple and practical approach based on clinical and pathological features.

## Vascular malformations

### Superficial capillary naevus

These pink, flat areas, composed of dilated capillaries in the superficial dermis (Figure 10.6), are found in at least 50% of neonates. The most common sites are the nape of the neck, forehead and glabellar region ('salmon patches' or 'stork marks') and the eyelids ('angel's kisses'). Most facial lesions fade quite quickly, but those on the neck persist, although often hidden by hair.

### Deep capillary naevus

'Port-wine stains' or 'port-wine marks' are formed by capillaries in the upper and deeper dermis. There may also be deeper components which may gradually extend over time.

Deep capillary naevi are less common but more cosmetically disfiguring than superficial lesions. Most occur on the head and neck and are usually unilateral, often appearing in the territory of one or more branches of the trigeminal nerve (Figure 10.7). They may be small or very extensive.

At birth, the colour may vary from pale pink to deep purple, but the vast majority of these malformations show no tendency to fade. Indeed they often darken with time, and become progressively thickened. Lumpy angiomatous nodules may develop.

These lesions are most unattractive, and patients often seek help. Modern lasers can produce reasonable results, and a range of cosmetics can be used as camouflage.

There are three important complications (see box).

---

**Complications of deep capillary naevus**

- An associated intracranial vascular malformation may result in fits, long-tract signs and learning disability. This is the Sturge–Weber syndrome
- Congenital glaucoma may occur when lesions involve the area of the ophthalmic division of the trigeminal nerve
- Growth of underlying tissues may be abnormal, resulting in hypertrophy of whole limbs—haemangiectatic hypertrophy

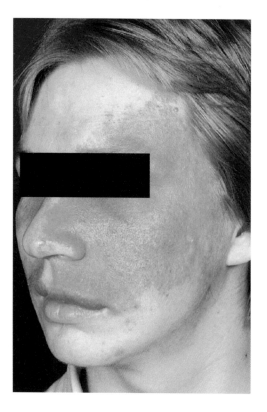

Figure 10.7 Deep capillary naevus ('port-wine stain').

If a deep capillary naevus is relatively pale, it may be difficult to distinguish from the superficial type, especially in the neonatal period. It is therefore wise always to give a guarded initial prognosis and await events.

## Childhood angiomas

These are quite distinct from pure vascular malformations in that they are characterized by the presence of actively growing and dividing vascular tissue, but some lesions are genuinely mixtures of malformation and angioma. Terminology can be difficult: 'strawberry naevus' and 'cavernous haemangioma' are still terms in common use, but we prefer simply to call them childhood or infantile angiomas.

The majority arise in the immediate postnatal period, but some are actually present at birth. They may appear anywhere, but have a predilection for the head and neck and the nappy area (Figure 10.8). Most are solitary, but occasionally there are more, or there are adjacent/confluent areas (called 'segmental' by some authorities). Lesions usually grow rapidly to produce dome-shaped, red–purple extrusions that may bleed if traumatized. The majority reach a maximum size within a few months. They may be large and unsightly.

Spontaneous resolution is the norm, sometimes beginning with central necrosis, which can look alarming. As a rule of thumb, 50% have resolved by age 5 and 70% by age 7. Some only regress partially and a few require plastic surgical intervention.

The management, in all but a minority, is expectant. It is useful to show parents a series of pictures of previous patients in whom the lesion has resolved

Specific indications for intervention:

1 If breathing or feeding is obstructed
2 If the tumour occludes an eye—this will lead to blindness (amblyopia)

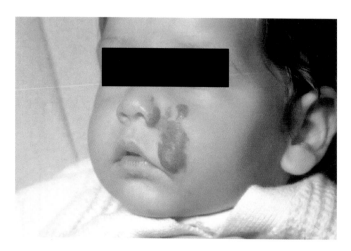

Figure 10.8 Cavernous haemangioma on the face.

**3** If severe bleeding occurs

**4** If the tumour remains large and unsightly after the age of 10

For many years, the mainstay of treatment for complications 1–3 has been high-dose prednisolone. This will almost always produce marked shrinkage, but may be replaced by propranolol which has very recently been reported to work even better. If these measures fail, and with persistent tumours, complex surgical intervention may be required.

### Rare angiomatous naevi

Rarely, infants are born with multiple angiomas of the skin and internal organs. This is known as neonatal or miliary angiomatosis and the prognosis is often poor.

## Other naevi

Naevi may develop from other skin elements, including connective tissue, mast cells and fat. For example, the cutaneous stigmata of tuberous sclerosis are connective tissue naevi (see Chapter 11), and the lesions of urticaria pigmentosa are mast cell naevi.

# 11

# Inherited disorders

*There is only one more beautiful thing than a fine healthy skin, and that is a rare skin disease.*
                    *Sir Erasmus Wilson, 1809–84*

A number of skin conditions are known to be inherited. Many are rare, and are therefore mentioned only briefly. There have been major advances in medical genetics in recent years, and the genes responsible for many disorders have been identified and their roles in disease clarified.

Several diseases in which genetic factors play an important part, such as atopic eczema, psoriasis, acne vulgaris and male-pattern balding, are described elsewhere in the book.

## The ichthyoses

The term 'ichthyosis' is derived from the Greek *ichthys*, meaning fish, as the appearance of the abnormal skin has been likened to fish scales. The ichthyoses are disorders of keratinization in which the skin is extremely dry and scaly (Figure 11.1). In most cases the disease is inherited, but occasionally ichthyosis may be an acquired phenomenon, e.g. in association with a lymphoma. There are several types of ichthyosis, which have different modes of inheritance (Table 11.1).

### Ichthyosis vulgaris (autosomal dominant ichthyosis)

This is the most common and is often quite mild. The scaling usually appears during early child-

*Lecture Notes: Dermatology*, 10th edition. © RAC Graham-Brown and DA Burns. Published 2011 by Blackwell Publishing Ltd.

hood. The skin on the trunk and extensor aspects of the limbs is dry and flaky, but the limb flexures are often spared. Ichthyosis vulgaris is frequently associated with an atopic constitution.

It has been demonstrated that loss-of-function mutations in the gene encoding for filaggrin (*FLG*) underlie ichthyosis vulgaris. The associated reduction of filaggrin leads to impaired keratinization. Loss-of-function mutations in *FLG* also strongly predispose to atopic eczema.

## X-linked recessive ichthyosis

This type of ichthyosis affects only males. The scales are larger and darker than those of dominant ichthyosis, and usually the trunk and limbs are extensively involved, including the flexures. Corneal opacities may occur, but these do not interfere with vision. Affected individuals are deficient in the enzyme steroid sulfatase—the result of abnormalities in its coding gene. Most patients have complete deletion of the steroid sulfatase gene, located on the short arm of the X-chromosome at Xp-22.3.

Both X-linked ichthyosis and autosomal dominant ichthyosis improve during the summer months.

## Ichthyosiform erythroderma and lamellar ichthyosis

A non-bullous form of ichthyosiform erythroderma (NBIE) is recessively inherited and is usually manifest at birth as a collodion baby appearance. Thereafter there is extensive scaling and redness. Lamellar ichthyosis is recessively inherited and affected infants also present as col-

Figure 11.1 Ichthyosis.

### Table 11.1 The ichthyoses

**Primary (congenital) ichthyosis**

Ichthyosis vulgaris (autosomal dominant ichthyosis)

X-linked recessive ichthyosis

Non-bullous ichthyosiform erythroderma

Bullous ichthyosiform erythroderma (epidermolytic hyperkeratosis)

Netherton's syndrome

Sjögren–Larsson syndrome

Refsum's disease

**Acquired ichthyosis**

Lymphoma

AIDS

Malnutrition

Renal failure

Sarcoidosis

Leprosy

lodion babies. Scaling is thicker and darker than in NBIE and there is less background erythema. These conditions are probably parts of a clinical spectrum caused by several different genes.

In bullous ichthyosiform erythroderma (epidermolytic hyperkeratosis), which is dominantly inherited, there is blistering in childhood and later increasing scaling until the latter predominates. There is a genetic defect of keratin synthesis involving keratins 1 and 10.

The ichthyosiform erythrodermas are all rare, as are some other ichthyosiform disorders, including Netherton's syndrome (ichthyosis linearis circumflexa and bamboo hair), Sjögren–Larsson syndrome (ichthyosis and spastic paraparesis), and Refsum's disease (ichthyosis, retinitis pigmentosa, ataxia and sensorimotor polyneuropathy).

## Acquired ichthyosis

When ichthyosis develops in adult life it may be a manifestation of a number of diseases, including underlying lymphoma, AIDS, malnutrition, renal failure, sarcoidosis and leprosy.

Treatment consists of regular use of emollients and bath oils. Urea-containing creams are also helpful. Oral retinoid treatment may be of benefit in the more severe congenital ichthyoses.

# Collodion baby

This term is applied to babies born encased in a transparent rigid membrane resembling collodion (Figure 11.2) (collodion is a solution of nitrocellulose in alcohol and ether used to produce a protective film/membrane on the skin after its volatile components have evaporated, and also employed as a vehicle for certain medicaments). The membrane cracks and peels off after a few days. Some affected babies have an underlying ichthyotic disorder whereas in others the underlying skin is normal. Collodion babies have increased transepidermal water loss, and it is important that they are nursed in a high humidity environment and given additional fluids.

Figure 11.2 Collodion baby.

# Palmoplantar keratoderma

Several rare disorders are associated with massive thickening of the horny layer of the palms and soles. The most common type is dominantly inherited. Many medical texts mention an association of palmoplantar keratoderma (tylosis) with carcinoma of the oesophagus—in fact this is extremely rare.

# Darier's disease (keratosis follicularis)

This is a dominantly inherited disorder that is usually first evident in late childhood or adolescence. It is caused by mutations in the *ATP2A2* gene at chromosome 12q23-24, which encodes an enzyme important in maintaining calcium concentrations in the endoplasmic reticulum. The abnormality results in impaired cell adhesion and abnormal keratinization.

The characteristic lesions of Darier's disease are brown follicular keratotic papules, grouped together over the face and neck, the centre of the chest and back, the axillae and the groins (Figure 11.3). The nails typically show longitudinal pink or white bands, with V-shaped notches at the free edges (Figure 11.4). There are usually numerous wart-like lesions on the hands (acrokeratosis verruciformis).

Figure 11.3 Darier's disease.

It is exacerbated by excessive exposure to sunlight, and extensive herpes simplex infection (Kaposi's varicelliform eruption) can occur.

Darier's disease responds to treatment with oral retinoids.

Figure 11.4 The nail in Darier's disease. note the longitudinal bands and V-shaped notching.

# Epidermolysis bullosa

This group of hereditary blistering diseases is described in Chapter 14.

# Ehlers–Danlos syndrome

There are a number of distinct variants of this condition, all of which are associated with abnormalities of collagen, principally defective produc-tion. The most common are dominantly inherited, but all types of Ehlers–Danlos syndrome are rare. Typical features are skin hyperextensibility and fra-gility, and joint hypermobility—some affected indi-viduals work as contortionists and 'India-rubber' men in circuses. In certain types there is a risk of rupture of major blood vessels because of defi-cient collagen in vessel walls.

# Tuberous sclerosis complex

Tuberous sclerosis complex (TSC) is the preferred name for what was previously known as tuberous sclerosis or epiloia (**epi**lepsy, **lo**w intelligence and **a**denoma sebaceum). It is a dominantly inherited disorder, but many cases are sporadic and repre-sent new mutations. In about half the cases the genetic abnormality occurs on chromosome 9q34 (TSC1) and in the others it is on chromosome 16p13 (TSC2).

There are hamartomatous malformations in the skin and internal organs. Characteristic skin lesions include: numerous pink papules on the face (Figure 11.5) (originally misleadingly called adenoma sebaceum), which are hamartomas of connective tissue and small blood vessels (angiofi-bromas); the 'shagreen' (having a resemblance to shark skin) patch on the back (a connective tissue naevus); periungual fibromas (Figure 11.6); and hypopigmented macules (ash leaf macules) which are best seen with the aid of Wood's light. The hypopigmented macules are often present at

Figure 11.5 Facial angiofibromas in tuberous sclerosis complex.

Figure 11.6 Periungual fibroma in tuberous sclerosis complex.

birth, but the facial lesions usually first appear at the age of 5 or 6. Affected individuals may have learning disabilities and epilepsy. Other features include retinal phakomas, pulmonary and renal hamartomas, and cardiac rhabdomyomas.

# Neurofibromatosis

There are two main forms of neurofibromatosis—type 1 (NF-1 or von Recklinghausen's disease) and type 2 (NF-2), both of which are of autosomal dominant inheritance. The gene for the more common type (NF-1) is located on chromosome 17q11.2 and that for NF-2 on chromosome 22q11.21. Both normally function as tumour-suppressor genes.

NF-1 is characterized by multiple café-au-lait patches, axillary freckling (Crowe's sign), numerous neurofibromas (Figure 11.7) and Lisch nodules (pigmented iris hamartomas). Other associated abnormalities include scoliosis, an increased risk of developing intracranial neoplasms, particularly optic nerve glioma, and an increased risk of hypertension associated with phaeochromocytoma or fibromuscular hyperplasia of the renal arteries.

NF-2 is characterized by bilateral vestibular schwannomas (acoustic neuromas), as well as other central nervous system tumours. It does not have significant cutaneous manifestations.

# Peutz–Jeghers syndrome

In this rare, dominantly inherited syndrome associated with mutations in a gene mapped to chromosome 19p13.3 there are pigmented macules (lentigines) in the mouth, on the lips, and on the hands and feet, in association with multiple hamartomatous intestinal polyps with low potential for malignant transformation.

# Hereditary haemorrhagic telangiectasia (Osler–Weber–Rendu disease)

This is a rare, dominantly inherited disorder in which numerous telangiectases are present on the face and lips, nasal, buccal and intestinal mucosae. Recurrent epistaxes are common, and there is also a risk of gastrointestinal haemorrhage. There is an association with pulmonary and cerebral arteriovenous fistulae. Visible vascular lesions can be treated with a laser.

# Basal cell naevus syndrome (Gorlin's syndrome)

Gorlin's syndrome is an autosomal dominant disorder associated with mutations of the tumour-suppressor gene *PTCH* on chromosome 9q22.3-3.1. Multiple basal cell carcinomas (BCCs) on the face and trunk are associated with characteristic palmar pits, odontogenic keratocysts of the jaw, calcification of the falx cerebri, skeletal abnormalities and medulloblastoma.

The BCCs should be dealt with when they are small. Radiotherapy is contraindicated because this promotes subsequent development of multiple lesions in the radiotherapy field.

# Gardner's syndrome

This condition is also dominantly inherited. The gene responsible is located on chromosome 5q21-

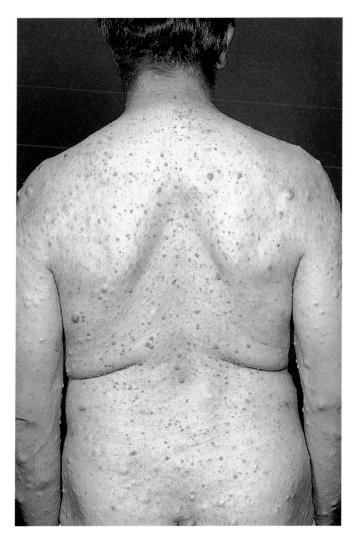

Figure 11.7 Von Recklinghausen's neurofibromatosis.

22, and it is thought that Gardner's syndrome and familial polyposis coli are allelic disorders caused by mutation in the *APC* (adenomatous polyposis coli) gene, which is another tumour-suppressor gene. Affected individuals have multiple epidermoid cysts, osteomas and large bowel adenomatous polyps that have a high risk of malignant change.

## Ectodermal dysplasias

These are disorders in which there are defects of the hair, teeth, nails and sweat glands. Most are extremely rare. One of the more common syn-dromes is hypohidrotic ectodermal dysplasia in which eccrine sweat glands are absent or markedly reduced in number, the scalp hair, eyebrows and eyelashes are sparse, and the teeth are widely spaced and conical. The absence of sweating causes heat intolerance. It is inherited as an X-linked recessive trait.

## Pseudoxanthoma elasticum

This recessively inherited abnormality is now thought to be a primary metabolic disorder in which *MRP6/ABCC6* gene mutations lead to metabolic abnormalities that result in progressive calcification of elastic fibres. This affects elastic tissue in the dermis, blood vessels and Bruch's membrane in the eye. The skin of the neck and axillae has a lax 'plucked chicken' appearance of tiny yellowish papules (Figure 11.8). Retinal angioid streaks, caused by ruptures in Bruch's membrane, are visible on fundoscopy (Figure 11.9). The abnormal elastic tissue in blood vessels may lead to gastrointestinal haemorrhage.

# Xeroderma pigmentosum

Ultraviolet (UV) damage to epidermal DNA is normally repaired by an enzyme system. In xeroderma pigmentosum, which is recessively inherited, this system is defective, and UV damage is not repaired. This leads to the early development of skin cancers. BCCs, squamous cell carcinomas and malignant melanomas may all develop in childhood. In some cases there is also gradual

Figure 11.8 'Plucked chicken' appearance of the skin in pseudoxanthoma elasticum.

Figure 11.9 Retinal angioid streaks in pseudoxanthoma elasticum (arrows).

neurological deterioration caused by progressive neuronal loss.

# Acrodermatitis enteropathica

In this recessively inherited disorder there is defective absorption of zinc. The condition usually manifests in early infancy as exudative eczematous lesions around the orifices, and on the hands and feet. Affected infants also have diarrhoea. Acrodermatitis enteropathica can be effectively treated with oral zinc supplements.

# Angiokeratoma corporis diffusum (Anderson–Fabry disease)

This condition is the result of an inborn error of glycosphingolipid metabolism. It is inherited in an X-linked recessive manner. Deficiency of the enzyme α-galactosidase A leads to deposition of ceramide trihexoside in a number of tissues, including the cardiovascular system, the kidneys, the eyes and peripheral nerves. The skin lesions are tiny vascular angiokeratomas that are usually scattered over the lower trunk, buttocks, genitalia and thighs. Associated features caused by tissue deposition of the lipid include those in the box.

---

**Anderson–Fabry disease**

- Premature ischaemic heart disease
- Renal failure
- Severe pain and paraesthesiae in the hands and feet
- Corneal and lens opacities

---

# Incontinentia pigmenti

An X-linked dominant disorder, incontinentia pigmenti occurs predominantly in baby girls, as it is usually lethal *in utero* in boys. Linear bullous lesions are present on the trunk and limbs at birth, or soon thereafter. The bullae are gradually replaced by warty lesions, and these in turn are eventually replaced by streaks and whorls of hyperpigmentation. The skin lesions follow Blaschko's lines. Incontinentia pigmenti is frequently associated with a variety of ocular, skeletal, dental and central nervous system abnormalities.

# Chromosomal abnormalities

Some syndromes caused by chromosomal abnormalities may have associated dermatological problems.

---

**Associated dermatological problems**

- Down's syndrome: increased incidence of alopecia areata and crusted scabies
- Turner's syndrome: primary lymphoedema
- Klinefelter's syndrome: premature venous ulceration
- XYY syndrome: premature venous ulceration; prone to develop severe nodulocystic acne

---

# 12

# Pigmentary disorders

*Bold was her face, and fair, and red of hew.*
*Chaucer,* The Wife of Bath

*The complexion of the skin and the colour of the*
*hair correspond to the colour of the moisture*
*which the flesh attracts—white, or red, or black.*
*Hippocrates*

## Introduction: normal pigmentary mechanisms

Our skin colour is important, and there are many references to it in prose and poetry. We all note skin colour in our initial assessment of someone, and cutaneous pigment has been used to justify all manner of injustices. Any departure from the perceived norm can have serious psychological effects and practical implications.

A number of factors give rise to our skin colour (see the box).

Normal pigmentary mechanisms have already been outlined in Chapter 1. Humans actually have a rather dull range of natural colours when compared with chameleons, peacocks, humming birds or parrots: normally only shades of brown and red. 'Brownness' is due to melanin, the intensity varying from almost white (no melanin) to virtually jet-black (lots). Melanin pigmentation is determined by simple mendelian principles: brown/black is autosomal dominant.

Red, on the other hand, is more complex genetically and is a bonus: only some people can produce phaeomelanin. Red is much more common in some races (e.g. Celts) than in others (e.g. Chinese).

Most human skin pigment is within keratinocytes, having been manufactured in melanocytes and transferred from one to the other in melanosomes. There are racial differences in production, distribution and degradation of melanosomes, but not in the number of melanocytes (see Chapter 1). There are, however, important genetic differences, reflected in the response to ultraviolet (UV) radiation, conventionally called 'skin types'.

---

**Skin colour factors**

- Haemoglobin
- Exogenous pigments in or on the skin surface
- Endogenously produced pigments (e.g. bilirubin)
- The pigments produced in the skin itself: melanin and phaeomelanin

The last two are the most important in dictating our basic skin colour

---

**Skin types**

- Type I: always burns, never tans
- Type II: burns easily, tans poorly
- Type III: burns occasionally, tans easily
- Type IV: never burns, tans easily
- Type V: genetically brown (e.g. Indian) or Mongoloid
- Type VI: genetically black (Congoid or Negroid)

---

*Lecture Notes: Dermatology*, 10th edition. © RAC Graham-Brown and DA Burns. Published 2011 by Blackwell Publishing Ltd.

The first response to UV radiation is an increased distribution of melanosomes. This rapidly increases basal layer pigmentation—the 'sun tan'. Tanning represents the skin's efforts to offer protection from the harmful effects of UV radiation, such as premature ageing and cancers. If solar stimulation is quickly withdrawn, as typically happens in a porcelain-white Brit after 2 weeks on the Costa del Sol, the tan fades rapidly and peels off with normal epidermal turnover. If exposure is more prolonged, melanin production is stepped up more permanently. We now look at states in which these pigmentary mechanisms appear to be abnormal, leading to decreased (hypo-) or increased (hyper-) pigmentation.

# Hypopigmentation

Among the most important causes of hypopigmentation are those in the box.

---

**Hypopigmentation causes**

**Congenital**

- Albinism
- Phenylketonuria
- Tuberous sclerosis complex
- Hypochromic naevi

**Acquired**

- Vitiligo
- Sutton's halo naevi
- Tuberculoid leprosy
- Pityriasis (tinea) versicolor
- Pityriasis alba
- Lichen sclerosus
- Drugs and chemicals:
  — occupational leukoderma
  — self-inflicted/iatrogenic
- Postinflammatory hypopigmentation

---

## Congenital

Some individuals are born with generalized or localized defects in pigmentation.

Albinism and phenylketonuria are due to genetic defects in melanin production. In albinos, the enzyme tyrosinase may be absent (tyrosinase negative), leading to generalized white skin and hair, and red eyes (the iris is also depigmented). Vision is usually markedly impaired, with nystagmus.

In some albinism, the enzyme is merely defective (tyrosinase positive). The clinical picture is not as severe, and colour gradually increases with age. However, skin cancers are very common in both forms. Albinism also illustrates the social importance of colour: in some societies, albinos are rejected and despised, in others they are revered.

The biochemical defect in phenylketonuria results in reduced tyrosine, the precursor of melanin, and increased phenylalanine (which inhibits tyrosinase). There is a generalized reduction of skin, hair and eye colour.

One of the cardinal signs of tuberous sclerosis complex (epiloia) is hypopigmented macules. These are often lanceolate (ash-leaf shaped), but may assume bizarre shapes. They are often the first signs of the disease. Any infant presenting with fits should be examined under Wood's light, as the macules can be seen more easily—see Chapter 2. Identical areas may occur without any other abnormality, when they are termed 'hypochromic naevi'.

## Acquired

Acquired hypopigmentation is common and, in darker skin, may have a particular stigma. This is partly because the cosmetic appearance is much worse, but also because white patches are inextricably linked in some cultures with leprosy. In olden times, all white patches were probably called leprosy: Naaman (who was cured of 'leprosy' after bathing in the Jordan [2 *Kings* 5:1–14]) probably had vitiligo (see below).

Vitiligo is the most important cause of patches of pale skin. The skin in vitiligo becomes depigmented and not hypopigmented, although as lesions develop this is not always complete.

Characteristically, otherwise entirely normal skin loses pigment completely (Figure 12.1). Patches may be small, but commonly become large, often with irregular outlines. Depigmentation may spread to involve wide areas of the body. Although vitiligo can occur anywhere, it is often strikingly symmetrical, involving the hands, and perioral and periocular skin.

The pathophysiology is poorly understood. Early on, melanocytes are still present, but produce no melanin. Later, melanocytes disappear completely, except deep around hair follicles. Vitiligo

Figure 12.1 A typical patch of vitiligo.

is generally thought to be an autoimmune process. Organ-specific autoantibodies are frequently present (as in alopecia areata, with which vitiligo may coexist).

Treatment is generally unsatisfactory. Topical steroids have their advocates, and psoralen and UVA (PUVA) can be successful. Cosmetic camouflage may be helpful. Sunscreens should be used in the summer, because vitiliginous areas will not tan and will burn easily.

In some patients, particularly children, areas repigment spontaneously. This is less common in adults and in longstanding areas. Repigmentation often begins with small dots coinciding with hair follicles. A similar appearance occurs in Sutton's halo naevus (see Chapter 10).

Tuberculoid leprosy is in the differential diagnosis of hypopigmentation, but the (usually solitary) patch of hypopigmented skin will also exhibit diminished sensation. Pale patches are also seen in the earliest stages: so-called 'indeterminate' leprosy.

The organism causing pityriasis versicolor (see Chapter 4) secretes azelaic acid. This results in hypopigmentation, most noticeably after sun exposure.

Pityriasis alba (a low-grade eczema) is a very common cause of hypopigmentation in children, especially in darker skins. Pale patches with a slightly scaly surface appear on the face and upper arms (Figure 12.2). The condition usually responds (albeit slowly) to moisturizers, but may require mild topical steroids. The tendency appears to clear at puberty.

Figure 12.2 Pityriasis alba on the cheek.

Lichen sclerosus (see Chapter 15) usually affects the genitalia. On other sites it is sometimes called 'white spot disease'.

Drugs and chemicals may cause loss of skin pigment. These may be encountered at work, but a more common source is skin lightening creams which, sadly, are all too commonly used by those with dark skin. The active ingredient is generally hydroquinone, which can be used therapeutically (see below).

Many inflammatory skin disorders leave secondary or postinflammatory hypopigmentation in their wake, due to disturbances in epidermal integrity and melanin production: both eczema and psoriasis often leave temporary hypopigmentation when they resolve. However, inflammation can destroy melanocytes altogether: in scars, after burns and in areas treated with cryo-therapy (it is the basis of the technique of 'freeze-branding').

# Hyperpigmentation

There are many causes of increased skin pigmentation, including excessive production of melanin, and the deposition in the skin of several other pigments, such as β-carotene, bilirubin, drugs and metals. The major causes are as shown in the box.

Figure 12.3 Café-au-lait patch in neurofibromatosis.

---

**Causes of hyperpigmentation**

**Congenital**

- Neurofibromatosis
- Peutz–Jeghers syndrome
- LEOPARD syndrome
- Incontinentia pigmenti

**Acquired**

- Urticaria pigmentosa
- Addison's disease
- Renal failure
- Haemochromatosis
- Liver disease
- Carotenaemia:
  — idiopathic
  — myxoedema
  — pernicious anaemia
- Acanthosis nigricans
- Chloasma
- Drugs and chemicals
- Postinflammatory hyperpigmentation

---

## Congenital

Hyperpigmentation is prominent in neurofibromatosis: café-au-lait marks (Figure 12.3) and axillary freckling are common. Speckled lentiginous pigmentation is seen around the mouth and on the hands in the Peutz–Jeghers syndrome, and similar but more widespread lentigines may accompany a number of congenital defects in the LEOPARD syndrome (**l**entigines, **e**lectrocardiographic abnormalities, **o**cular hypertelorism, **p**ulmonary stenosis, **a**bnormalities of the genitalia, **r**etardation of growth and **d**eafness.).

Incontinentia pigmenti is a rare congenital disorder that causes hyperpigmentation in a whorled pattern, following a phase of blisters and hyperkeratotic lesions, and sometimes accompanied by other congenital abnormalities.

## Acquired

Urticaria pigmentosa (which is due to abnormal numbers of dermal mast cells) is most common in children, but may affect adults. There is a widespread eruption of indistinct brown marks which urticate if rubbed.

Chloasma, or melasma, is more common in women than men. Characteristically, hyperpigmentation develops on the forehead, cheeks and chin (Figure 12.4). Provoking factors include sunlight, pregnancy and oestrogen therapy, but chloasma may occur spontaneously. Treatment is difficult. Avoidance of precipitating factors (especially sunlight and oestrogens where possible) may help. Topical hydroquinone preparations are sometimes used.

Various drugs and chemicals cause cutaneous hyperpigmentation (see Chapter 21).

In postinflammatory hyperpigmentation, disruption of the epidermis results in deposition of melanin granules in the dermis (pigmentary incontinence). Many skin disorders do this, particularly in pigmented skin, but lichen planus is particularly troublesome. There is no useful treatment, but the pigmentation gradually fades with time.

Figure 12.4 Typical chloasma.

Hyperpigmentation is an important physical sign in several systemic diseases:

1 Addison's disease: the changes are most marked in skin creases, scratch marks and the gums
2 Renal failure: may cause muddy-brown skin colour
3 Haemochromatosis: causes a deep golden-brown hue, diabetes and liver disease
4 Some chronic liver diseases, e.g. primary biliary cirrhosis

β-Carotene (a yellow pigment) accumulates harmlessly in the skin in some normal individuals who ingest large amounts of carrots and orange juice (rich sources). The colour is most marked on the palms and soles. Similar deposition is seen in some patients with myxoedema and pernicious anaemia.

Another important, although rare, cause of acquired hyperpigmentation is acanthosis nigricans. This may or may not be associated with a systemic disease (see Chapter 19).

# 13

# Disorders of the hair and nails

*If a woman have long hair, it is a glory to her.*
*St Paul (1 Corinthians, 11:15)*

*The hair takes root in the head at the same time as the nails grow.*

*Hippocrates*

## Introduction

St Paul clearly understood the importance of a good head of hair to human well-being and Hippocrates (see above) knew that hair and nails were intimately connected. There are conditions that affect both or either alone. We deal with abnormalities of hair first and then nail disorders, but there is some overlap.

## Hair abnormalities

Abnormalities of hair and nails may be the result of:

1 Local factors
2 Generalized skin disease
3 Systemic disease

Hair is important psychologically. Disturbances in growth or physical characteristics, even of minor degree, may be very upsetting: did Kojak really like being bald? Remember that the distress caused

*Lecture Notes: Dermatology*, 10th edition. © RAC Graham-Brown and DA Burns. Published 2011 by Blackwell Publishing Ltd.

is not necessarily proportionate to the severity apparent to an observer.

Patients present with three main hair abnormalities:

1 Changes in physical properties (e.g. colour or texture)
2 Thinning or loss of hair
3 Excessive hair growth, including growth in abnormal sites

## Changes in physical properties of scalp hair

Common physical changes that are seen in hair are as follows:

---

**Physical changes to hair**

**Pigmentation—greying/whiteness**
- Genetic diseases, e.g. albinism, phenylketonuria
- Premature greying:
  - physiological
  - pathological, e.g. pernicious anaemia
- Ageing
- Vitiligo
- Alopecia areata

**Textural abnormalities**
- Brittleness
- Coarseness
- Curliness

## Change in colour

Greying of the hair, whether or not premature, is permanent, including, usually, the white hair in scalp vitiligo. Regrowing hair in alopecia areata (see below) is often white initially, but repigments later.

## Textural abnormalities

Brittleness or coarseness may accompany hair thinning in hypothyroidism and iron deficiency (see below). Hair may also become lack-lustre from hairdressing techniques (back-combing, bleaching and drying). In men, hair may become curly in the early stages of androgenetic alopecia (see below).

## Scalp hair loss

## Congenital disorders

Abnormal scalp hair loss is a feature of some congenital disorders.

---

**Congenital disorders and scalp hair loss**

- Ectodermal dysplasias
- Premature ageing syndromes
- Monilethrix
- Pili torti
- Marie–Unna alopecia
- Disorders of amino acid metabolism
- Scalp naevi (especially epithelial or organoid)
- Aplasia cutis

---

Very few of these conditions are treatable, but they require careful assessment, including microscopic examination of hair shafts.

## Acquired disorders

Patients most commonly seek advice about hair loss when it is from the scalp, although other areas may be affected. The most effective approach to the diagnosis of acquired scalp hair loss is:

1 to consider whether the changes are diffuse or circumscribed
2 to assess the state of the scalp skin.

When this information is combined with some knowledge of the disorders mentioned below, a preliminary diagnostic assessment can be made.

Telogen effluvium is often triggered by major illness, operations, accidents or other stress. A large percentage of hairs suddenly stop growing, enter the resting or 'telogen' phase, and start to fall out about 3 months later. Therefore, ask about any major upset in the appropriate period. Pull gently on hairs on the crown or sides, and several will come out easily: with a hand lens, the bulb looks much smaller than normal. Telogen effluvium should settle spontaneously, but can unmask androgenetic alopecia (see below), and some patients find that their hair never returns completely to normal.

Appropriate tests will exclude important systemic diseases, and correct treatment may restore hair growth.

---

**Acquired causes of scalp hair loss**

**Diffuse hair loss with normal scalp skin**
- Telogen effluvium
- Thyroid disease
- Iron deficiency
- Drugs
- Systemic lupus erythematosus
- Secondary syphilis
- Alopecia totalis

**Androgenetic alopecia**

**Circumscribed hair loss with normal scalp skin**
- Alopecia areata
- Traction
- Trichotillomania

**Hair loss with abnormal scalp skin**
*Without scarring*
- Severe psoriasis or seborrhoeic dermatitis
- Tinea capitis (see Chapter 4)

*With scarring*
- Discoid lupus erythematosus
- Lichen planus
- Pseudopelade
- Cicatricial pemphigoid
- Lupus vulgaris

---

Many drugs can induce hair loss.

---

**Drugs inducing hair loss**

- Cytotoxic agents
- Antithyroid agents, especially thiouracil
- Anticoagulants
- Retinoids
- Thallium

---

All of these processes can be confused with alopecia areata (see below) when the latter is widespread and rapidly progressive.

Androgenetic alopecia (or common balding) occurs in both men and women. It is due to the effects of androgens in genetically susceptible individuals.

In men, the process may begin at any age after puberty, but is much more common from the 30s onwards. By age 70, 80% of men show some hair loss. Hair is usually lost first at the temples and/or on the crown, but there may be complete hair loss, sparing a rim at the back and sides. Terminal hairs become progressively finer and smaller, until only a few vellus hairs remain. The extent and pace of this vary widely.

In women, the process is slower and less severe, but causes much distress. Up to half of all women have mild hair loss on the vertex by age 50 and, in some, more severe thinning occurs. There may be accompanying hirsutism (see below).

Until recently there was no known treatment, but early use of topical minoxidil may help both men and women, and relatively selective antiandrogenic agents (e.g. finasteride) are becoming available.

## Circumscribed hair loss with normal scalp skin

### Alopecia areata

The cause of this disorder is unknown but it is probably an autoimmune process. As in vitiligo (see Chapter 12), organ-specific autoantibodies (to thyroid, adrenal or gastric parietal cells) are often found in patients' sera.

*History*: one or more areas of baldness suddenly appear on the scalp, in the eyebrows, beard or elsewhere. It is most common in childhood and early adult life, although periodic recurrences may happen at any age.

*Examination*: patches are typically round or oval (Figure 13.1); the skin usually appears completely normal, although there may be mild erythema; a number of areas may develop next to each other, giving rise to a moth-eaten appearance; close examination of the edge of a patch reveals the pathognomonic feature—'exclamation mark hairs'—short hairs that taper towards the base (Figure 13.2).

*Prognosis*: most patches regrow after a few weeks but further episodes are common; initial hair growth may be white; occasionally, the process spreads and may become permanent—if this involves the whole scalp it is termed alopecia

Figure 13.1 A typical patch of alopecia areata.

Figure 13.2 The edge of the area seen in Figure 13.1. Exclamation mark hairs are visible at the margin.

Figure 13.3 Traction alopecia.

totalis and if the whole body is affected, the name alopecia universalis is applied. The nails may be affected in severe cases (see below).

*Treatment*: this is difficult, but topical and intralesional steroids may help. Calcineurin inhibitors are used, and topical sensitization with agents such as diphencyprone is also used.

Chronic traction may cause circumscribed alopecia, especially around scalp margins (Figure 13.3). It is seen in young girls with tight ponytails, Sikh boys and African–Caribbean children whose hair is dressed in multiple little pigtails.

In trichotillomania, hair is pulled, twisted or rubbed out, and affected site(s) are covered in broken hairs of different lengths. There may be psychological factors (see Chapter 20).

## Hair loss with abnormal scalp skin

Psoriasis, seborrhoeic dermatitis and other inflammatory processes can cause temporary hair loss: an important cause is tinea capitis (see Chapter 4).

In some conditions, fibrosis accompanies the inflammation, and this may result in permanent damage to hair follicles, and obvious loss of tissue or atrophy. This is known as scarring or cicatricial alopecia.

Examination of the rest of the skin may provide important clues.

**Causes of cicatricial alopecia**

**Discoid lupus erythematosus**
- Prominent plugging of the hair follicles
- Look for lesions on the face

**Lichen planus**
- May accompany lichen planus elsewhere
- Nail involvement is common (see Chapter 15)

**Cicatricial pemphigoid**
- Alopecia follows blistering

**Lupus vulgaris (cutaneous tuberculosis)**

**Trigeminal trophic syndrome**
- May follow herpes zoster because of hypoaesthesia and chronic trauma

**Pseudopelade**
- Small patches of scarring alopecia without distinguishing features

In most of these conditions, a biopsy is essential. In cases where lupus erythematosus or cicatricial pemphigoid is suspected, immunofluorescence should also be performed.

## Generalized hair loss

Generalized hair loss is rare, but may accompany endocrine disturbances, especially hypothyroidism or hypopituitarism. Drugs, particularly cytotoxics, may induce widespread alopecia. As has been mentioned, alopecia areata may lead to complete hair loss—alopecia universalis.

## Excessive hair and hair in abnormal sites

### Hirsutism

This term is applied to excessive growth of hair in a female, distributed in a male secondary sexual pattern.

A search for more serious causes is indicated if the changes are of rapid onset.

**Causes of hirsutism**

- Mild hirsutism is quite common in elderly women
- It may be a genetic trait in younger females, when the changes may accompany a general reduction in scalp hair (see Androgenetic alopecia)
- Minor endocrine disturbances, especially polycystic ovary syndrome
- Drugs with androgenic activity
- Virilizing tumours

Treatment includes shaving, waxing, depilatory creams, electrolysis and laser ablation. The antiandrogen cyproterone acetate may help.

## Hypertrichosis

Excessive hair growth in a non-sexual distribution may occur in both sexes. There are several causes:

**Causes of hypertrichosis**

- Congenital generalized, e.g. Cornelia de Lange syndrome
- Congenital localized, e.g. 'faun-tail' in spina bifida occulta
- Drugs such as:
  — minoxidil (now used for baldness—see above)
  — ciclosporin
  — hydantoins
  — systemic steroids
- Anorexia nervosa
- Cachexia
- Porphyria cutanea tarda: associated with scarring and milia
- Pretibial myxoedema: overlying plaques

# Nail abnormalities

Nail changes may be non-specific, or characteristic of specific processes. They may occur in isolation, but the nails are abnormal in several disorders.

## Disorders with abnormal nails

### Congenital

- Especially disorders of keratinization, e.g. Darier's disease
- Ectodermal dysplasias
- Due to scarring, e.g. dystrophic epidermolysis bullosa

### Acquired

- Psoriasis
- Eczema/dermatitis
- Lichen planus
- Alopecia areata/totalis
- Fungal infections

## Common nail abnormalities

### Brittleness

- Increases with age
- Seen in iron deficiency (see also Koilonychia) and thyroid disease

### Roughness (trachyonychia)

- Common and often non-specific
- May result from widespread pitting (see below)

### Beau's lines

- Horizontal grooves that follow a major illness

### Pits

- Classic feature of psoriasis
- Severe alopecia areata (smaller, more evenly distributed than in psoriasis)
- Eczema/dermatitis (coarse dents and irregular pits)

### Onycholysis

- Lifting of nail plate off nail bed
- Causes:
  - psoriasis
  - fungal infection (see Chapter 4)
  - thyrotoxicosis
  - space-occupying lesion (e.g. exostosis or tumour)
- May be no other identifiable abnormality present

### Clubbing

- Sign of pulmonary, liver or thyroid disease; may be familial

### Discoloration

- White marks—common normal variant
- White nails—associated with cirrhosis
- Pale—anaemia
- Half red/half pale—renal disease
- Sulfur yellow—fungal infection
- Uniform yellow—'yellow nail syndrome' (bronchiectasis and lymphoedema)
- Green–blue—*Pseudomonas* infection
- Brown–black—melanoma, haematoma
- Linear brown—naevus

### Koilonychia

- Nails with a concave upper surface (spoon-shaped)
- Causes:
  - iron deficiency
  - inherited

### Washboard nails (Figure 13.4)

- Habitual picking of nail fold leads to surface ridging

### Onychogryphosis

- Grossly thickened, distorted nails (Figure 13.5) often due to neglect

### 'Pterygium'

- Damage leads to epithelium encroaching on nail surface
- Most common cause—lichen planus

### Loss of nails

- Causes:
  - pterygium
  - scarring, e.g. Stevens–Johnson syndrome
  - severe inflammation, e.g. pustular psoriasis

Figure 13.4 'Washboard' nails on the thumbs: the result of a habit tic.

Figure 13.5 Onychogryphosis.

## Common disorders of the paronychium

Patients may complain of disorders of the area around the nail—the paronychium.

### Paronychia

There are two common forms: acute and chronic. In acute paronychia, an abscess in the nail fold forms, points and discharges. It is nearly always staphylococcal. Chronic paronychia is discussed in Chapter 4.

### Ingrowing nails

Over-curved nails (especially on big toes) dig into the lateral nail fold, leading to chronic inflammation and overproduction of granulation tissue. Sometimes this can be prevented by trimming nails straight, but surgical intervention is often required.

### Periungual warts

Warts are discussed in Chapter 3. Periungual warts are unsightly and extremely difficult to eradicate.

Figure 13.6 (a) Myxoid cyst of the finger; (b) Insertion of a needle releases crystal-clear, gelatinous contents.

## Myxoid cyst

Small cystic swellings may appear on the proximal nail fold (Figure 13.6). The nail may develop a linear depression. Clear gelatinous fluid can be expressed, if the surface is breached (Figure 13.6b).

These cysts are more common in middle-aged and elderly people. A myxoid cyst is essentially a ganglion connected to the distal interphalangeal joint by a narrow pedicle. Treatment is with cryotherapy, or various surgical procedures.

# 14

# Bullous disorders

*All that blisters is not pemphigus.*
*Graham-Brown and Burns, 1990*

## Causes

The skin has a limited repertoire of changes, but few are more dramatic than an eruption of blisters or bullae. There are many causes.

This is a fairly comprehensive differential diagnostic list for further reading. Some disorders, such as impetigo and the viral causes, are mentioned elsewhere in this book; this chapter deals with the most important remaining causes of blistering.

### Causes of bullae

**Physical injury**
- Cold, heat, friction
- Severe oedema

**Infections (see Chapters 3 and 4)**

*Bacterial*
- Impetigo

*Viral*
- Chickenpox
- Herpes zoster
- Herpes simplex
- Smallpox and vaccinia
- Hand, foot and mouth disease

*Fungal*
- Tinea pedis with pompholyx

**Arthropods (see Chapter 5)**
- Insect bites

**Drugs (see also Chapter 21)**
- Barbiturates, sulfonamides, iodides, furosemide, nalidixic acid (light induced)
- Drug-induced pemphigus and pemphigoid
- Fixed drug eruptions

**Skin disorders**

*Congenital*
- Epidermolysis bullosa

*Acquired*
Bullae are a major feature in:
- Pemphigus
- Bullous pemphigoid
- Cicatricial pemphigoid
- Dermatitis herpetiformis
- Linear IgA disease
- Epidermolysis bullosa acquisita
- Toxic epidermal necrolysis

Bullae may occur in:
- Erythema multiforme (Stevens–Johnson syndrome)
- Eczema (including pompholyx)
- Lichen planus
- Psoriasis (pustular)
- Vasculitis

**Metabolic disease**
- Porphyria cutanea tarda
- Diabetes mellitus

*Lecture Notes: Dermatology*, 10th edition. © RAC Graham-Brown and DA Burns. Published 2011 by Blackwell Publishing Ltd.

## Physical causes of bullae

Burns due to cold, heat or chemical injury may cause blisters, as may extreme friction (e.g. the feet of vigorous squash players or joggers).

## Oedema

Tense bullae may arise in severe oedema of the lower legs.

## Arthropods

Remember that insect bites very commonly present as tense bullae (see Chapter 5). In the UK, this is most common in late summer and early autumn (fall).

## Drugs

Several drugs cause blistering (see above). Blisters caused by nalidixic acid occur on the lower legs after sun exposure. Fixed drug eruptions may blister (see Chapter 21).

## Skin disorders

Primary skin disorders giving rise to bullae may be congenital or acquired. In some, bullae are an integral part of the clinical presentation. In others, blisters are a less prominent or constant feature, and the reader should consult the appropriate chapter for further information.

## Congenital

### Epidermolysis bullosa

Although very rare, this is an important group of disorders. Babies are born with fragile skin that blisters on contact. There are several variants, with splits at different levels in the skin; all are unpleasant and some are fatal.

Diagnosis requires sophisticated investigation, including electron microscopy to determine the level of the blister.

The differential diagnosis of blistering in a neonate must also include a number of other disorders:

1 Impetigo (pemphigus neonatorum)
2 Staphylococcal scalded skin syndrome (see below)
3 Incontinentia pigmenti (see Chapter 11)

## Acquired

### Pemphigus

The cardinal pathological processes in all forms of pemphigus are:

1 A split within the epidermis
2 Loss of adhesion of epidermal cells ('acantholysis')

These changes may be just above the basal layer (pemphigus vulgaris; Figure 14.1) or higher in the epidermis (pemphigus foliaceus; Figure 14.2).

The most common variant is pemphigus vulgaris, which presents with flaccid blisters and erosions (Figure 14.3). These may be anywhere, but in over 50% of patients the mouth is affected (Figure 14.4), and perineal lesions are also com-

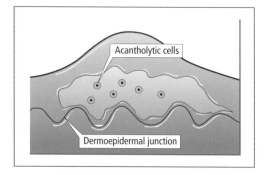

**Figure 14.1** Pemphigus vulgaris: split just above the basal layer, with overlying acantholysis of epidermal cells.

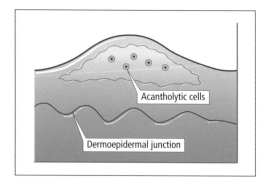

**Figure 14.2** Pemphigus foliaceus: similar changes to those in Figure 14.1 but higher in the epidermis.

Figure 14.3 Pemphigus vulgaris: flaccid blisters and erosions.

Figure 14.4 Pemphigus: oral erosions.

mon. The blisters rupture easily and the resulting erosions heal very slowly, if at all. A highly characteristic feature is the Nikolsky sign: skin at the edge of a blister slides off when pushed by a finger or picked up with forceps. This is only seen in pemphigus and toxic epidermal necrolysis (see below). Pemphigus vegetans is a variant of pemphigus vulgaris in which vegetating masses occur, especially in the flexures.

Pemphigus foliaceus does not always present with obvious blisters, because they are even more fragile than in pemphigus vulgaris: there may only be non-specific scaly areas, and scalp and face involvement can closely simulate seborrhoeic eczema. One variant known as pemphigus erythematosus remains localized to the face, and may be confused with lupus erythematosus.

**Investigations**

The investigations performed in all forms of pemphigus are the same:

1 Biopsies from involved skin, preserving an early blister (intact if possible) for histopathology
2 Perilesional tissue for direct immunofluorescence
3 Serum for indirect immunofluorescence

The immunopathology of pemphigus vulgaris and foliaceus is identical:

1 Bright staining around epidermal cells with antibodies directed against immunoglobulin G (IgG) and C3 (Figure 14.5)
2 Circulating antiepithelial antibody (in most patients)

Figure 14.5 Pemphigus: direct immunofluorescence. IgG is found around epidermal cells.

## Treatment

Treatment must be vigorous. Before the advent of systemic corticosteroids, most patients died, often after a long and debilitating illness.

High doses of prednisolone (60–120 mg daily) are used. The dose is gradually reduced when new blistering has ceased (usually in about 4–6 weeks). Immunosuppressive agents such as azathioprine, chlorambucil, cyclophosphamide or methotrexate, and the monoclonal antibody, rituximab, are useful in reducing systemic steroid dosage. Good nursing and metabolic management are crucial because pemphigus patients may be systemically ill. Widespread erosions cause loss of protein and fluid, and secondary infection is common. If the mouth is severely involved, patients cannot eat and may become severely catabolic.

## Bullous pemphigoid and cicatricial pemphigoid

Bullous pemphigoid is much more common than pemphigus. More than 80% of patients are aged over 60.

Bullae are the key feature, but are not always present initially. The process may begin with a non-specific phase known as 'pre-pemphigoid', characterized by intense irritation and well-defined, slightly elevated, erythematous areas.

When bullae develop they are usually numerous, tense, dome shaped and may be filled with blood (Figure 14.6). They vary from a few millimetres to several centimetres in diameter, often arising on urticated erythema as well as on normal skin. Although lesions may appear anywhere, there is a predilection for the limbs. Oral involve-

Figure 14.6 Bullous pemphigoid: numerous tense blisters.

ment may occur. When blisters burst, healing is usually rapid. Some blisters do not burst, and the fluid is simply reabsorbed. Scarring is rare, but there is a distinctive variant, characterized by marked scarring, known as cicatricial pemphigoid. This condition has a predilection for oral, conjunctival and genital epithelium.

The diagnosis in both forms of pemphigoid requires:

1 A biopsy for histopathology
2 A biopsy for direct immunofluorescence
3 Serum for indirect immunofluorescence is a much less valuable investigation and is often omitted

The pathological findings are as shown in the box.

---

**Pathological findings in pemphigoid**

- A subepidermal blister (Figure 14.7)
- A linear band of IgG and C3 at the basement membrane zone (Figure 14.8): this is attached to an antigen in the area of the hemidesmosomes and anchoring fibrils
- A circulating IgG antibody to basement membrane is found in 70% of patients with bullous pemphigoid but the titre is of no significance
- No circulating antibody in cicatricial pemphigoid

---

**Treatment**
Both variants require treatment with systemic steroids, in moderate doses, usually with immunosuppressives such as azathioprine or chlorambucil.

Bullous pemphigoid generally responds rapidly, and maintenance therapy with small doses is usually possible. The condition appears to be self-limiting in some. Cicatricial pemphigoid is much less responsive.

## Dermatitis herpetiformis

Dermatitis herpetiformis is uncommon. Its importance lies in its ability to cause severe itching, and its association with gluten-sensitive enteropathy.

Clinically, the cardinal features are a history of intense pruritus and grouped erythematous papules and vesicles, most typically on the elbows (Figure 14.9) and extensor surfaces of the forearms, knees and shins, buttocks, shoulders and scalp.

Itching often results in excoriations and secondary eczematization; it is not always possible to find intact vesicles or bullae.

Dermatitis herpetiformis should be considered in any patient with severe itching and

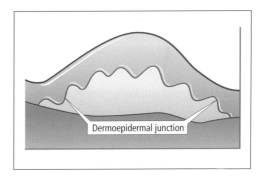

Figure 14.7 Bullous pemphigoid: the split is subepidermal.

Figure 14.8 Bullous pemphigoid: direct immunofluorescence. IgG at the basement membrane zone.

Figure 14.9 Dermatitis herpetiformis: the elbow is a typical site.

inflammatory skin changes in the distribution mentioned above.

The diagnosis requires:

1 A biopsy of a blister or, preferably, a new pink papule for histopathology
2 A biopsy of normal skin for immunofluorescence
3 A jejunal biopsy

The main pathological findings are as shown in the box.

---

**Pathological findings in dermatitis herpetiformis**

- A subepidermal blister that is indistinguishable, when fully formed and intact, from that seen in bullous pemphigoid
- However, in very early prevesicular lesions (hence the pink papule), or at the edge of a vesicle, there are small neutrophil 'microabscesses' in dermal papillary tips (Figure 14.10). These are pathognomonic
- Granular IgA in the dermal papillary tips on immunofluorescence (Figure 14.11)
- There are no circulating antibodies
- Gut changes of gluten sensitivity, ranging from increased lymphocyte numbers to various grades of villous atrophy

---

**Treatment**

Dermatitis herpetiformis responds dramatically to sulfones. Dapsone is the drug of first choice but it induces haemolysis, especially at higher doses. Alternatives are sulfapyridine and sulfamethoxypyridazine (unfortunately, these can sometimes be difficult to obtain). A gluten-free diet is essential, not only because the condition may be controlled by diet alone, but because there may be an increased risk of gut lymphoma (similar to coeliac disease).

## Linear IgA disease

Occasionally, patients with a pemphigoid- or dermatitis herpetiformis-like presentation are found

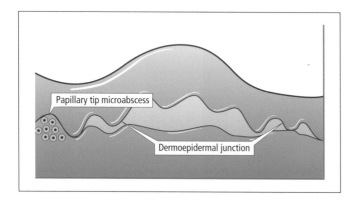

Papillary tip microabscess

Dermoepidermal junction

Figure 14.10 Dermatitis herpetiformis: papillary tip microabscesses as well as a subepidermal blister.

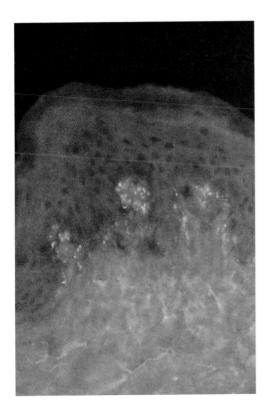

Figure 14.11 Dermatitis herpetiformis: immunofluorescence of normal skin. Granular deposits of IgA in dermal papillae.

to have a linear band of IgA at the basement membrane on immunofluorescence. This is now generally considered to be a separate bullous disease, which may be seen in both children and adults.

Often the blisters are arranged in rows or clusters (a 'string of pearls').

# Rarer blistering diseases

## Porphyria cutanea tarda

This is rare, but presents as small blisters and erosions on the backs of the hands, and on the forearms and face, following sun exposure or minor trauma. In most patients there is an underlying liver disorder, and often alcohol abuse. It may be triggered by drugs, notably oestrogens.

## Toxic epidermal necrolysis

This is a term applied to an acute disorder in which there is loss of the epidermis, usually over wide areas of the body surface (Figure 14.12), although localized forms have been described. The Nikolsky sign is positive. Primary toxic epidermal necrolysis is usually an adverse reaction to a drug.

Extensive epidermal loss leads to severe dehydration and protein depletion. Patients require intensive care, and are best managed in a manner similar to those with burns.

## Bullous erythema multiforme (Stevens–Johnson syndrome)

This is a reactional state due to a wide variety of triggers (see Chapter 15). In severe erythema multiforme, bullae may be the most prominent clinical feature.

Figure 14.12 Severe skin loss in toxic epidermal necrolysis.

# 15

# Miscellaneous erythematous and papulosquamous disorders, and light-induced skin diseases

*Miscellaneous: of mixed composition or character; of various kinds; many-sided.*
                    Concise Oxford English Dictionary

This chapter is a mixed bag: it covers a number of common and/or important skin disorders that have not found a place elsewhere.

## Urticaria and angioedema

Urticaria is the clinical term for a group of disorders characterized by the formation of weals—swellings of the skin that disappear leaving no visible sign. Most of us have experienced one common form—after falling (or being pushed) into nettles (the term 'nettle-rash' is used commonly for urticaria). The main pathological change

*Lecture Notes: Dermatology*, 10th edition. © RAC Graham-Brown and DA Burns. Published 2011 by Blackwell Publishing Ltd.

is dermal oedema due to vascular dilatation, often in response to histamine (and probably other mediators) released from mast cells. In some patients, there are also small numbers of lymphocytes, indicating an autoimmune aetiology.

### Clinical features

The skin itches or stings; weals develop, white at first, then pink with a white rim; lesions can become very extensive and appear in many sites at once, but *always* clear spontaneously within a few hours, even though new lesions may continue to develop.

Typical lesions of urticaria are shown in Figure 15.1.

A frequent accompanying feature of urticaria is angioedema, in which oedema extends into subcutaneous tissues, especially around the eyes, the lips, and in the mouth and pharynx. The swelling may be alarming, occasionally resulting in complete closure of the eyes, swelling of the lips and tongue, and compromise of the airway.

Figure 15.1 Urticaria.

Urticaria and angioedema may form part of a systemic anaphylactic reaction.

## Clinical forms of urticaria and angioedema

### Acute urticaria

Attacks last only a few hours or days. Common causes include the following:

1 Contact with plants (e.g. nettles), animal fur (e.g. dogs, cats, horses) or foods (e.g. milk, egg-white)
2 Ingestion of foods, especially nuts, shellfish and strawberries
3 Ingestion of drugs, e.g. aspirin and penicillin

People who have atopy (with asthma, eczema or hay fever) are more susceptible. The reaction is generally triggered by immunoglobulin E (IgE) antibodies; some reactions, e.g. to aspirin, are due to direct mast cell degranulation.

## Chronic urticaria

Attacks last for weeks, months or years. Contrary to popular expectations, a single causative factor is rarely found. Chronic ingestion of food colourings and preservatives may occasionally be important, but in most patients chronic urticaria is due to an autoimmune process or to one of the physical stimuli discussed below.

## The physical urticarias

Several physical insults may trigger urticarial responses:

1 Dermographism: weals appear after scratch-marks (Figure 15.2); this may occur alone or with other forms of urticaria
2 Pressure (delayed): weals develop up to 24h after pressure is applied
3 Cholinergic urticaria: affects young men; sweating is accompanied by small white weals with a red halo on the upper trunk

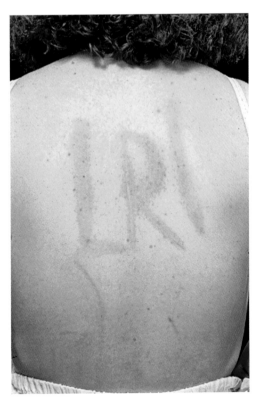

Figure 15.2 Dermographism.

**4** Cold: contact with any cold object or blasts of cold air induce the formation of weals
**5** Water
**6** Sunlight
**7** Heat

## Hereditary angioedema

In this very rare autosomal dominant condition:

**1** C1 esterase inhibitor is lacking or defective
**2** There are sudden attacks of angioedema that can be life threatening
**3** The gut may be affected, giving rise to spasms of abdominal pain

## Urticaria pigmentosa

Abnormal accumulations of mast cells result in multiple pigmented macules that cause urticaria on being rubbed (see also Chapter 12).

## Urticaria in systemic disease

An urticarial eruption may be part of a systemic disorder, especially hepatitis B.

## Treatment of urticaria

If a possible trigger can be elicited from the history, it should be avoided. Aspirin, and aspirin-like substances, should be avoided by anyone prone to urticaria.

Most types of urticaria respond to $H_1$-receptor antihistamines, although some of the rarer physical forms do not. A large range of agents is available, many of which cause central nervous system (CNS) depression, but several newer antihistamines have little or no sedative effect (e.g. desloratadine, levocetirizine, fexofenadine). These are now drugs of first choice. It may help to add an $H_2$-receptor antagonist (cimetidine, ranitidine), but this is controversial.

It is sometimes necessary to use other agents, such as systemic steroids, ciclosporin and adrenaline (see below).

---

**Management of urticaria**

- Acute attacks: a few days' treatment is usually sufficient
- Chronic urticaria: give a dose of antihistamine which suppresses the eruption completely; maintain this dose for several months; gradually withdraw treatment
- Angioedema: may require parenteral therapy with adrenaline, antihistamines and steroids
- Anaphylaxis: adrenaline is required
- Hereditary angioedema: does not respond to antihistamines or steroids; danazol works by increasing levels of the missing enzyme; purified enzyme preparations are available for acute attacks

---

# Erythema multiforme

The classic lesion of erythema multiforme is the 'iris' or 'target' lesion (Figure 15.3): a round or oval

Figure 15.3 'Target' lesions of erythema multiforme.

area of erythema, with a dusky, purplish centre. Sometimes the centre becomes paler and a blister forms.

## History

Lesions appear suddenly, enlarge over the course of a few days and fade (often leaving pigmentary disturbances). The whole process settles in about 3 weeks. Repeated episodes are rare, but can be triggered by herpes simplex virus (see below).

## Aetiology

Erythema multiforme may occur out of the blue, but there are several recognized triggers.

---

**Triggers for erythema multiforme**

- Herpes simplex virus: the most common trigger; as herpes may be recurrent, so may herpes-related erythema multiforme
- Other viruses: orf, hepatitis, mumps
- Radiotherapy
- Cancers
- Connective tissue diseases
- A wide variety of drugs

---

## Examination

The distribution characteristically includes extensor surfaces of the arms and legs, but most important diagnostically is involvement of the palms and soles.

## Pathology

The histological changes are at the dermoepidermal junction and may represent a delayed hypersensitivity reaction.

## Treatment

Erythema multiforme is self-limiting, and treatment is not usually required.

## Stevens–Johnson syndrome

At its most extreme, erythema multiforme causes a major systemic disturbance. There is an acute onset, with severe inflammation of conjunctivae, mouth and genitalia (Figure 15.4), which may prevent normal eating, affect micturition and cause ocular scarring. Patients occasionally die of severe bronchopulmonary involvement or renal failure.

## Treatment

Close attention must be given to fluid balance and nutrition. The role of systemic steroids is controversial, because the morbidity from steroids probably outweighs that from the disease.

---

# Exfoliative dermatitis (erythroderma)

These terms (either will do) are used to describe a state in which most of the skin becomes red, inflamed, oedematous and scaly (Figure 15.5).

The correct management depends on the underlying disease process, because the optimum

Figure 15.4 Erosions on the lips in bullous erythema multiforme.

Figure 15.5 Exfoliative dermatitis.

treatment is different. The following are the four most important causes of exfoliative dermatitis:

1 Psoriasis
2 Eczema/dermatitis
3 Drug reactions
4 Lymphomas (especially cutaneous T-cell lymphoma)

### Clinical features

These are generally the same, regardless of the underlying cause: the skin is red, hot and scaly; there may be generalized lymphadenopathy; there is a loss of control of temperature regulation, and there are bouts of shivering as the body attempts to compensate for heat loss by generating metabolic heat.

### Effects

Cardiac output is increased, protein is lost from the skin (and the gut), water loss from the skin is increased, patients radiate heat into their surroundings, there is a rise in metabolic rate, with mobilization of energy sources and increased muscle activity, and the body cannot compensate for long, especially in elderly patients.

### Complications

Cardiac failure; renal failure; sudden death due to central hypothermia.

### Treatment

1 Stop any potential causative drugs (see Chapter 21)
2 Nurse the patient in a warm room
3 Attend to secondary medical problems (e.g. dehydration, heart failure and infections)
4 Biopsy the skin to obtain a definitive diagnosis
5 Give a short course of systemic steroids (if the diagnosis is known to be psoriasis from the outset, commence systemic anti-psoriatic drugs as well as or instead of the steroids —see Chapter 8)
6 Initiate appropriate treatment for underlying diagnosis

# Lichen planus

Lichen planus is a rather variable disorder, said to affect 1% of new referrals to a dermatologist. The most common pattern is an acute eruption of itchy papules (Figure 15.6).

### Sites of predilection

Wrists, ankles and the small of the back, mouth and genitalia.

### Clinical features

1 Skin lesions:
  (a) flat-topped
  (b) shiny
  (c) polygonal (Figure 15.6)
2 Surface: fine network of dots or lines called 'Wickham's striae'
3 Colour: 'violaceous' (reddish-purple)
4 Oral: lacy, reticulate streaks on the lining of the cheeks (Figure 15.7), gums and lips

Figure 15.6 (a) Typical papules of lichen planus and (b) papules of lichen planus on the wrist—a classic site.

Figure 15.7 Oral lesions in lichen planus.

In most patients, the eruption settles over a period of a few months. There are a number of variants, some of which are more persistent.

## Aetiology

Lichen planus is a T-cell-mediated attack on the epidermis, similar changes being seen in graft-versus-host reactions. However, the cause of lichen planus in most instances remains a mystery.

---

**Variants of lichen planus**

- Hypertrophic: lichenified lumps appear on the legs
- Atrophic: largely seen in the mouth, lesions may be very chronic; small risk of carcinoma
- Follicular: may result in permanent scarring and hair loss
- Nail disease: nail changes may be very slight, or may lead to complete nail loss
- Drug induced: see Chapter 21

---

## Treatment

Potent topical steroids usually suppress irritation; very extensive or severe oral disease may need systemic steroids or ciclosporin.

Figure 15.8 Characteristic appearance of vulval lichen sclerosus.

---

# Lichen nitidus

Probably a variant of lichen planus, this uncommon disorder produces clusters of tiny, asymptomatic papules.

---

# Lichen sclerosus

Lichen sclerosus (previously called lichen sclerosus et atrophicus) is a disorder of unknown aetiology.

## Sites of predilection

The genitalia, especially in women.

## Clinical features

1 White, atrophic patches on the vulva, perineum and perianal skin (Figure 15.8), or glans penis and foreskin

2 Similar plaques may develop elsewhere
3 Purpura and blistering may appear
4 Vulval lichen sclerosus easily becomes eroded and haemorrhagic, with severe soreness and irritation

## Complications

Vulvovaginal stenosis; development of squamous cell carcinoma.

## Childhood disease

Lichen sclerosus in prepubertal girls often presents with dysuria and pain on defecation. It may be misdiagnosed as sexual abuse, but lesions are usually easy to diagnose, and parents and child can be reassured. The prognosis of childhood disease is good, as many clear at puberty.

## Disease in males

Lichen sclerosus may be seen on the glans and prepuce (sometimes called 'balanitis xerotica obliterans'), and can give rise to phimosis and meatal stenosis. A significant number of boys undergo circumcision because of phimosis due to lichen sclerosus. There is a risk of squamous cell carcinoma. Extragenital lesions may also occur.

### Treatment

The disease in adults generally pursues a chronic relapsing course. Very potent topical steroids provide symptomatic relief in vulval disease, and clobetasol propionate is the treatment of choice. Patients should be kept under surveillance because of the risk of neoplastic change.

# Pityriasis rosea

Pityriasis rosea is a self-limiting disorder, predominantly affecting children and young adults.

### Clinical features

1 There may be a mild prodromal illness
2 One or more 'herald patches' appear. A herald patch is large, red, oval and scaly, and usually appears on the trunk or upper arm (often misdiagnosed, especially as ringworm!)
3 A few days later, there is a sudden eruption of pink, oval patches on the trunk, upper arms and thighs

There are three especially notable features:

1 On the trunk, lesions largely lie with their long axes in lines sweeping from the back to the front (almost as if they were following spinal nerves). This is said to resemble an 'inverted

Figure 15.9 Pityriasis rosea.

Christmas tree' (Figure 15.9)—but that depends on your image of a Christmas tree! However, once understood, this sign will never be forgotten and *no other disorder produces this*
2 The scale on the surface of each lesion peels from the centre towards the edge, resulting in a so-called 'peripheral collarette' (Figure 15.10)
3 If the diagnosis has still not been made, it becomes clear when the rash disappears (as it always does) in 6–8 weeks

Figure 15.10 Pityriasis rosea: the 'peripheral collarette' of scale.

## Treatment

Usually unnecessary, but mild topical steroids may help to relieve irritation.

## Atypical pityriasis rosea

There may be no gap between the herald patch and the generalized rash; the eruption may extend down the arms and legs, and occasionally spares the trunk altogether; lesions may be so numerous that the distribution described above is not apparent; the inflammation may be so intense that it causes blisters.

# Pityriasis lichenoides

Small brownish-red papules surmounted by a 'plate' of scale appear on the trunk and limbs. Some patients have more acutely inflamed lesions that heal to leave pockmarks.

# Pityriasis rubra pilaris

Pityriasis rubra pilaris (PRP) occurs in localized or generalized forms. All types are rare. Lesions are reddish-orange, and hair follicles are prominently involved. Generalized change is a very rare cause of exfoliative dermatitis (see above).

# Miliaria or 'prickly heat'

This is the exotic name for little red bumps that some people develop in hot humid conditions. It is due to sweat duct obstruction. It should not be confused with polymorphic light eruption (see below), which is often erroneously called prickly heat, but in which the lesions are induced by light *not* heat. The condition is also seen in infants, particularly in the nappy area.

# Pregnancy rashes

Pregnancy may alter the course of a number of skin disorders, such as acne, eczema, psoriasis and vulval warts, and it may trigger erythema multiforme.

There are also three important conditions related to pregnancy itself.

---

**Conditions related to pregnancy**

**Pruritus of pregnancy**
- Up to 20% of women; may be due to oestrogen-induced cholestasis

**Polymorphic eruption of pregnancy**
- Blotchy, urticarial and papular rash with intense itching
- Onset in third trimester
- Lesions favour abdomen
- Particular predilection for striae (Figure 15.11)
- Fades shortly after delivery

**Herpes (pemphigoid) gestationis**
- Blisters on urticated background
- Variant of bullous pemphigoid
- Rare

---

# Light-induced skin disease

*But yet the light that led astray*
*Was light from Heaven*
                    *Robert Burns*, The Vision

Sunlight is generally thought to be beneficial: adverts for sunbeds, solaria and foreign holidays all bear witness to this twentieth-century obsession. However, ultraviolet (UV) radiation (especially in excess) initiates, wholly or in part, many unwanted skin changes:

- Some are chronic: cancers and keratoses (see Chapter 9); the yellowing, coarsening and wrinkling known as 'photoageing'. Note that most of today's tanned beauties are tomorrow's wrinkled prunes!
- Some are more acute: sunburn; reactions to a combination of plants or drugs and light
- Some are due to metabolic disturbances, whereas in others the cause is quite unknown
- UV radiation may also exacerbate certain pre-existing skin disorders (see below)

Figure 15.11 Polymorphic eruption of pregnancy.

## Sunburn

Most of us are familiar with sunburn, even if only in others. Excessive medium-wavelength UV radiation induces erythema and, if severe, blistering. The dose required depends on skin type (see Chapter 12), and the intensity of the UV radiation: skin types I and II are very prone to sunburn; sunlight around midday is the most intense.

Treatment of established sunburn is difficult, but calamine lotion and topical steroids may help symptomatically. Prevention is much better than cure.

Sun care should include avoidance of intense exposure, hats and clothing, sunglasses and sunscreens. Exposed surfaces should be covered as far as possible. Sunscreens come in a range of potencies, graded by sun protection factor (SPF) number. This number indicates the approximate multiple of time to redness that the agent will provide: if the exposure time to redness is normally 10 min, SPF 6 sunscreen will prolong this to about an hour.

## Polymorphic light eruption

Frequently misdiagnosed as 'prickly heat' (see above), this affects women more often than men, and typically trouble starts in adolescence or early adulthood.

### Clinical features

An eruption develops on light-exposed surfaces, most commonly the face, arms, legs and the 'V' of the neck. Individual lesions vary from papules to plaques. Blisters are sometimes seen. The reaction may occur only in very strong sunlight, but even mild British summer sunshine can be the trigger.

### Treatment

Preseason PUVA (psoralen and UVA) is helpful. Antimalarials may be of some benefit, and sunscreens and clothing will help prevent the eruption.

## Actinic prurigo

Actinic prurigo is a rare disorder of childhood in which eczematous areas develop on the face and

---

**Unwanted cutaneous reactions to light**

- Sunburn
- Polymorphic light eruption
- Solar urticaria (see above)
- Actinic prurigo
- Juvenile spring eruption
- Hydroa vacciniforme

- Photosensitive eczema
- Porphyrias
- Pellagra
- Xeroderma pigmentosum
- Phytophotodermatitis
- Drug reactions

backs of the hands every summer, and disappear in the winter. The cause is unknown, and attempted treatment is often ineffective.

## Juvenile spring eruption

Little boys occasionally develop blisters on the ears in spring, and this is given the grand title of 'juvenile spring eruption'. It is probably a variant of polymorphic light eruption.

## Photosensitive eczema and chronic actinic dermatitis

Some individuals develop eczema of light-exposed surfaces. In others, a pre-existing eczema becomes much worse on exposure to light.

One cause is a contact dermatitis to airborne chemicals, such as perfumes or plant extracts (e.g. chrysanthemums). A similar picture may occur with drugs.

The changes tend to become more intense until the skin is permanently thickened and inflamed. This state is termed 'chronic actinic dermatitis'.

### Treatment

This is very difficult. Barrier sunscreens containing titanium may help, and azathioprine has been shown to be of benefit.

## Porphyrias

This miscellaneous group of disorders is due to a variety of enzyme defects in the haem production pathways. Some, but not all, are associated with photosensitivity.

The most common in northern Europe is erythropoietic protoporphyria, in which burning in the sun (even through glass) develops in early childhood. A form known as 'variegate porphyria' is seen in some Dutch and South African pedigrees.

It is perhaps worth mentioning that one of the rarest porphyrias (congenital erythropoietic porphyria or Günther's disease) may be the origin of the werewolf legend. Sufferers become disfigured, hairy and anaemic (hence the werewolf's craving for blood). They avoid sunlight because of severe photosensitivity (the werewolf prowls at night when the moon is full—a logical time to prowl if there is no other source of illumination!).

## Pellagra

A photosensitive rash in malnourished individuals should suggest pellagra. In western societies the classic triad of diarrhoea, dermatitis and dementia is seen only in people with alcohol problems and those who are reclusive.

## Xeroderma pigmentosum

This rare disorder often presents with photosensitivity in early childhood (see also Chapter 11).

## Phytophotodermatitis

Every summer, we see patients who have developed a rash after contact with plants on sunny days. Linear, streaky dermatitis (Figure 15.12) results, and residual pigmentary disturbances are common. One important cause is giant hogweed, but there are several others.

Figure 15.12 A phytophotodermatitis.

## Light-induced drug reactions

Several groups of drugs are associated with photoallergic and phototoxic reactions (see Chapter 21).

## Disorders exacerbated by light

A number of disorders may show a deterioration or provocation on exposure to light. The mechanisms for this are unclear.

---

**Disorders exacerbated by light**

- Lupus erythematosus
- Rosacea
- Psoriasis
- Darier's disease
- Herpes simplex

# 16

# Vascular disorders

## Leg ulcers

By far the most common type of leg ulcer is the venous ulcer (varicose ulcer; gravitational ulcer). Other causes of leg ulceration include ischaemia, vasculitis, skin neoplasia and certain haematological disorders.

### Venous leg ulcers

Venous return from the legs is dependent on the deep and superficial venous systems and activity of the calf muscles. When the calf muscles contract they pump blood in the deep veins towards the heart against gravity. Valves in the deep veins prevent reflux of blood when the muscles relax. During relaxation of the calf muscles blood passes from the superficial veins into the deep veins via the saphenofemoral and saphenopopliteal junctions and numerous perforating veins. If the valves in the deep veins are incompetent the calf muscle pump cannot function effectively and venous hypertension develops. Congenital abnormalities of the venous system, and valve damage after deep vein thrombosis, contribute to incompetence. Genetic factors are important because certain racial groups have a low prevalence of venous hypertension and venous ulcers.

The high pressure in the deep veins of the legs is transmitted via incompetent perforating veins to the superficial venous system (resulting in 'varicose' veins), and eventually to the capillary network. Skin capillaries become dilated and tortuous, and there is increased transudation of fluid into the surrounding tissues. Fibrinogen in the transudate is converted to fibrin, which forms cuffs around blood vessels. Transfer of oxygen and nutrients to the surrounding tissues is impeded, and the relatively ischaemic tissues are susceptible to ulceration, either spontaneously or after minor trauma. This 'fibrin cuff' theory is only one of the proposed mechanisms for tissue ischaemia in venous hypertension, and the pathomechanics of ulceration have not been fully elucidated.

Problems caused by venous hypertension usually occur in middle or old age, and women, particularly if obese, are predominantly affected. The clinical features are as follows.

> **Venous hypertension: clinical features**
>
> - Varicose veins
> - Oedema
> - Lipodermatosclerosis
> - Hyperpigmentation
> - Eczema
> - Atrophie blanche
> - Ulceration

### Lipodermatosclerosis

This term refers to areas of induration, caused by fibrosis, on the lower parts of the legs, above the ankles (Figure 16.1). There is initially an area of erythema, and this subsequently becomes purple–brown in colour. On palpation, affected areas feel indurated. When the process is circumferential the tissues around the ankle are constricted and the leg above is oedematous, producing the classic 'inverted champagne bottle' appearance.

*Lecture Notes: Dermatology*, 10th edition. © RAC Graham-Brown and DA Burns. Published 2011 by Blackwell Publishing Ltd.

Figure 16.1 Lipodermatosclerosis.

Figure 16.2 Atrophie blanche.

## Hyperpigmentation

Haemosiderin, derived from red cells extravasated from dilated, leaky capillaries, produces areas of brown discoloration.

## Eczema

Areas of 'varicose' eczema are common.

## Atrophie blanche

This term is applied to areas of scar tissue within which are prominent dilated capillaries. Scattered pink dots are seen on a white background (Figure 16.2). Such areas are very prone to ulcerate, and the ulcers are usually extremely painful.

## Ulcers

The most common site for a venous ulcer is the medial aspect of the leg, just above the medial malleolus (Figure 16.3), but the lateral malleolar area may also be affected.

Rarely, a squamous cell carcinoma may develop in a longstanding venous ulcer (Marjolin's ulcer).

## Treatment

Varicose eczema may be treated with mild potency topical steroids. Colour Doppler duplex sonography should be performed, and assessment by a vascular surgeon is an important aspect of management, as some patients benefit significantly from surgery on incompetent superficial veins. In addition, it is essential to assess the arterial supply in patients with leg ulcers because they may have a remediable arterial abnormality. It is not uncommon to discover both venous and arterial pathology in individuals with leg ulcers.

Another essential component of the management of venous ulcers is reduction of venous hypertension and oedema by compression bandaging, which improves calf muscle pump function and opposes gravitational venous reflux. It is vital, however, to establish that the arterial supply to a limb is adequate (by assessing the ankle–brachial pressure index (ABPI) and by Doppler studies) before using compression bandaging.

Figure 16.3 Venous ulcer.

Secondary infection, often with a mixed bacterial flora, occurs in most venous ulcers. However, systemic antibiotic therapy is not necessary unless there is associated cellulitis (see Chapter 3).

There are numerous agents that have been marketed as topical therapies for leg ulcers, including alginate, hydrogel and hydrocolloid dressings, but a simple regimen of regular irrigation with saline and the application of a low adherence dressing is adequate in many cases, if combined with compression bandaging. The most important concept to remember is that, unless an effort is made to deal with the primary problem by compression bandaging and vein surgery when indicated, it doesn't matter what magical agent is applied to the ulcer because it won't heal.

When a venous ulcer has healed it is important to maintain compression by wearing appropriate compression hosiery.

## Ischaemic ulcers

Ischaemic ulceration is usually a manifestation of atherosclerotic peripheral vascular disease. Typically, ischaemic ulcers occur on the dorsum or the sides of the foot, between the toes, or on the heel, in an individual with a history of intermittent claudication and, later, rest pain. There are usually associated risk factors such as smoking, hypertension and diabetes. Pedal pulses are reduced or absent, and Doppler studies will demonstrate impaired blood flow. Ischaemic ulcers are usually painful.

The advice of a vascular surgeon should be sought.

## Vasculitic ulcers

Vasculitis associated with a number of disorders, including rheumatoid arthritis and systemic lupus erythematosus (SLE), may produce leg ulcers.

## Neoplastic ulcers

Basal cell carcinomas and squamous cell carcinomas arising on the legs may resemble, and be mistaken for, venous ulcers. However, they usually occur above the ankle region. If there is any suspicion that an ulcer is neoplastic, a biopsy should be performed.

## Haematological disorders and leg ulcers

Uncommon causes of leg ulcers include hereditary spherocytosis, sickle cell anaemia and thalassaemia. The mechanism of ulceration in these conditions is related to tissue hypoxia due to blockage of skin capillaries by abnormally shaped red cells.

---

# Vasculitis

Vasculitis is an inflammatory process affecting blood vessels. There have been several attempts at classification of vasculitis and none has proved entirely satisfactory, but systems employed are usually based on the size of vessel involved and the histological features. One proposed classification has two major categories—small and larger vessel vasculitides. The size of vessel involved in the process provides an indication of the accompanying systemic features, in that vasculitis affecting small vessels is associated with glomerulonephritis whereas larger vessel vasculitis is associated with arterial aneurysms and renovascular hypertension.

Factors involved in the pathogenesis of vasculitis include immune complexes, in which the antigens are of bacterial, viral or drug origin, antineutrophil cytoplasm antibodies (ANCAs) and various cytokines. Clinically, vasculitis may present as urticaria, livedo reticularis, purpuric papules, nodules, haemorrhagic bullae or ulcers.

Evaluation of a patient with suspected vasculitis should include pathological confirmation of the clinical diagnosis (skin biopsy for histology and direct immunofluorescence), assessment of the extent of the disease (involvement of internal organs, especially the presence of proteinuria/haematuria) and an attempt to establish the underlying aetiology (full blood count, antinuclear antibodies [ANAs], ANCAs, viral titres, antistreptolysin-O titres, chest radiographs).

---

### Classification

**Small vessels**

- Cutaneous small vessel vasculitis (leukocytoclastic vasculitis)
- Henoch–Schönlein purpura
- Drug-induced vasculitis
- Urticarial vasculitis

**Larger vessels**

- Polyarteritis nodosa
- Wegener's granulomatosis
- Nodular vasculitis
- Temporal arteritis

---

# Clinical presentations of vasculitis

## Small vessel

### Cutaneous small vessel vasculitis (leukocytoclastic vasculitis)

This is the most common type of vasculitis encountered in dermatology, and in current classifica-

tions cutaneous small vessel vasculitis (CSVV) is a term applied to any patient with small vessel vasculitis of the skin. Typically, the patient presents with numerous palpable, purpuric lesions on the legs, predominantly below the knees (Figure 16.4). Some lesions may develop into haemorrhagic vesicles or bullae. Histologically, there is fibrinoid necrosis of small blood vessels, and a perivascular infiltrate composed predominantly of neutrophil polymorphs. The perivascular tissues also contain extravasated red cells, and fragments of polymorph nuclei (nuclear dust). These changes are initiated by deposition of immune complexes in small vessels, complement activation and production of polymorph chemotactic factors. Polymorphs attracted to the area release enzymes that damage the vessel wall. Drugs, or bacterial or viral infections may act as the antigenic triggering factor, but often the initiating factor is not discovered.

In many cases there is no evidence of involvement of any organ other than the skin, but, if CSVV is accompanied by features suggesting a systemic vasculitis, such as myalgia, arthralgia, proteinuria, haematuria, abdominal pain and gastrointestinal haemorrhage, then the diagnostic label should be reassessed, because CSVV is a feature of other vasculitides, including Henoch–Schönlein purpura and Wegener's granulomatosis.

### Treatment

If a trigger can be identified, then it should be eliminated. A period of bed rest and treatment with non-steroidal anti-inflammatory drugs often result in complete resolution of the skin lesions. Colchicine and dapsone may be of benefit in some cases.

## Henoch–Schönlein purpura

Henoch-Schönlein purpura (HSP; anaphylactoid purpura) is the name given to a systemic small vessel vasculitis that occurs predominantly in children and is associated with deposition of IgA immune complexes in the skin (palpable purpura on the elbows, knees and buttocks), joints (arthritis), kidneys (glomerulonephritis) and gastrointestinal tract (abdominal pain and gastrointestinal haemorrhage). Perivascular IgA deposits are characteristic of HSP.

Upper respiratory tract infections often precede HSP.

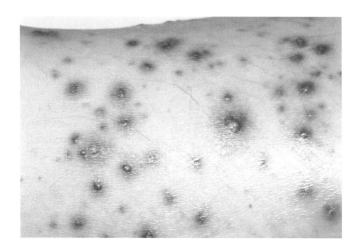

Figure 16.4 Cutaneous small vessel vasculitis.

## Treatment

Systemic steroid therapy is of benefit, particularly for nephritis, and in patients with severe renal disease other immunosuppressive agents may be required.

## Drug-induced vasculitis

Many drugs can be responsible for vasculitis, often of immune-complex-mediated leukocytoclastic type, but other patterns occur (see Chapter 21).

## Urticarial vasculitis

The appearance is similar to that of urticaria but differs in that individual lesions last longer than 24 h and often have a purpuric component. Although it is associated with a number of disorders it is a particular feature of connective tissue diseases, predominantly Sjögren's syndrome and SLE.

## Larger vessel

## Polyarteritis nodosa

Also known as periarteritis nodosa, this is an uncommon type of necrotizing vasculitis that affects medium-sized arteries throughout the body. Patients with polyarteritis nodosa (PAN) often have underlying infection with organisms that include the hepatitis B virus. Manifestations include pyrexia, weight loss, arthralgia and myalgia. The most significant clinical sign is the presence of cutaneous or subcutaneous nodules along the course of superficial arteries. Vessel

Figure 16.5 Erythema nodosum.

damage results in aneurysm formation. Livedo reticularis and skin ulceration are other features. There may be renal, gut, cardiac and nervous system involvement.

There is a type of PAN that affects the skin alone. Livedo reticularis and cutaneous nodules occur on the legs, usually below the knees.

## Treatment

High-dose steroid therapy is used in cases not associated with hepatitis B. Patients with hepatitis B-associated PAN are treated with a combination of an antiviral agent and an immunosuppressant. Cutaneous PAN usually responds to small doses of systemic steroids.

## Wegener's granulomatosis

This is a rare form of necrotizing granulomatous vasculitis affecting principally arteries of the respiratory tract, and associated with glomerulonephritis. Skin lesions take the form of palpable purpura and tender subcutaneous nodules on dependent areas. It is associated with the presence of ANCAs.

## Nodular vasculitis

The antigenic trigger for this form of vasculitis, which occurs predominantly in middle-aged women, is probably a bacterial infection of some type, but in many cases the precise aetiology is not discovered. Inflammatory nodules, produced by a vasculitis in the deep dermis and subcutaneous fat, occur on the legs. These may ulcerate. Other organs are not involved.

## Temporal arteritis (giant cell arteritis)

Skin changes are rare, but ulceration may occur on the temporal and parietal regions of the scalp.

# Other disorders involving blood vessels

## Erythema nodosum

This condition usually affects children and young adults, and is characterized by the development of multiple, tender, erythematous nodules, usually on the shins (Figure 16.5), but occasionally also on the forearms. As each nodule regresses it changes colour from red to purple to yellow-green—like a fading bruise. Pathologically, erythema nodosum is an inflammatory process of fat (panniculitis).

It is thought to be a hypersensitivity reaction triggered by the causes in the box.

> **Causes**
>
> - Streptococcal infection
> - Drugs, particularly sulfonamides
> - Sarcoidosis
> - Primary tuberculosis
> - Inflammatory bowel disease
>
> In some cases no precipitating factor is discovered

Investigation of a patient with erythema nodosum should include culture of a throat swab, antistreptolysin titre, chest radiograph and tuberculin skin test.

## Treatment

In most cases bed rest and simple analgesia are all that is required. The lesions will gradually resolve over a period of a few days.

## Behçet's disease

The principal features of this disorder are recurrent, severe oral and genital ulceration, and uveitis. Skin lesions include erythema nodosum and pustules at sites of minor trauma such as venepuncture sites.

## Pyoderma gangrenosum

See Chapter 19.

## Perniosis (chilblains)

Chilblains are painful, inflammatory lesions provoked by exposure to cold. The most common sites for chilblains are the fingers and toes, but they may also occur on fatty prominences such as the fat pads on the medial aspects of the knees, and on the thighs. A characteristic type of chilblains occurs on the lateral aspects of the thighs of female horse riders (Figure 16.6)—this is related to the chill factor produced by galloping along in the middle of winter. 'Chilblains' is a

Figure 16.6 Chilblains on the thigh in a keen horsewoman.

rather unimpressive word, so dermatologists call this disorder 'equestrian cold panniculitis'.

Treatment for chilblains is not very satisfactory. The best management is prophylaxis, by wearing warm gloves and thick socks, and, in the case of the equestrian, thermal underwear and clothing made of modern insulating materials.

# 17

# Connective tissue diseases

## Lupus erythematosus

Lupus erythematosus is an autoimmune disorder that occurs in two main forms—discoid lupus erythematosus (DLE), in which the skin alone is affected, and systemic lupus erythematosus (SLE), which affects both the skin and the internal organs. A small proportion of patients with DLE may subsequently develop SLE. A third variant, subacute cutaneous lupus erythematosus (SCLE), is characterized by distinctive skin lesions that may be associated with systemic features.

The pathogenesis of lupus erythematosus has not been fully elucidated, but probably involves a combination of genetic factors predisposing to autoimmunity, and environmental agents such as viral and bacterial antigens acting as triggering factors.

### Discoid lupus erythematosus

Classically, DLE affects light-exposed areas—principally the face and neck, but also the dorsa of the hands and the arms. Lesions may be precipitated or exacerbated by sunlight. Individual lesions consist of scaling, erythematous plaques, with prominent follicular plugging. If the scale is lifted off, follicular plugs may be seen on its

undersurface—the so-called 'carpet-tack' (or 'tin-tack') sign. There may be only a few lesions, but extensive, cosmetically disfiguring involvement of the facial skin can occur. Lesions heal with scarring, and the typical picture is of an active, erythematous scaly margin enclosing a central area of scarred, hypopigmented, atrophic skin (Figure 17.1). The scalp may be involved, producing areas of scarring alopecia in which follicles are permanently destroyed. Occasionally, the buccal or nasal mucosae are affected.

### Investigations

The diagnosis can be confirmed by skin biopsy. Histology shows a periadnexal lymphocytic infiltrate, liquefaction degeneration of the basal layer of the epidermis, follicular plugging and hyperkeratosis. Direct immunofluorescence of lesional skin reveals granular deposits of IgG and/or IgM at the dermoepidermal junction.

### Treatment

Potent fluorinated topical steroids are helpful in many cases, but, if they are ineffective, intralesional injection of triamcinolone or oral therapy with the antimalarial hydroxychloroquine may be required. In severe extensive disease oral steroids may be of benefit. Light-exposed areas should be protected by a sunscreen with a high sun protection factor (SPF). Where there is extensive

*Lecture Notes: Dermatology*, 10th edition. © RAC Graham-Brown and DA Burns. Published 2011 by Blackwell Publishing Ltd.

Figure 17.1 Discoid lupus erythematosus.

Figure 17.2 Facial erythema in systemic lupus erythematosus.

involvement of facial skin, the use of cosmetic camouflage can be of benefit.

## Systemic lupus erythematosus

This is a multisystem disorder that may affect the skin, joints, heart and pericardium, lungs, kidneys, brain and haematopoietic system. Typically, the disease affects women, particularly of childbearing age, and progresses in a series of exacerbations and remissions.

Mucocutaneous lesions include oropharyngeal ulceration, diffuse alopecia, Raynaud's phenomenon, vasculitis and photosensitivity. Often there is facial erythema in a 'butterfly' distribution (Figure 17.2). The 'butterfly' is represented by erythema on the cheeks linked by a band of erythema across the nose. However, by far the most common cause of this pattern of facial erythema is rosacea (see Chapter 6).

Systemic manifestations include those in the box.

---

**Manifestations of systemic lupus erythematosus**

**Polyserositis**
- Arthralgia and arthritis (usually non-erosive)
- Pericarditis
- Pleurisy with effusions

**Nephritis**

**Central nervous system involvement**
- Psychosis and convulsions

**Haematopoietic abnormalities**
- Haemolytic anaemia
- Leukopenia
- Thrombocytopenia

**Pyrexia, weight loss and general malaise**

## Investigations

These should include a full blood count (FBC) and biochemistry, complement levels, urinalysis, ECG (electrocardiograph) and chest radiograph.

A number of autoantibodies may be found in individuals with SLE. Antinuclear antibodies (ANAs) at high titre are found in most patients with SLE, and anti-double-stranded DNA antibodies (anti-dsDNA) are characteristic. Others include anti-Ro (also known as anti-SSA) and anti-La (anti-SSB), which are associated with neonatal lupus, and antiphospholipid antibodies. A positive rheumatoid factor and biological false-positive serological tests for syphilis may also be found.

Direct immunofluorescence of involved skin shows the same pattern of immunoglobulin deposition seen in DLE (see above).

## Treatment

Systemic steroids and immunosuppressive agents are the mainstay of treatment. Light-exposed areas of skin should be protected by sunscreens with a high SPF.

## Subacute cutaneous lupus erythematosus

In this 'subset' of lupus, non-scarring, papulosquamous or annular lesions occur predominantly on light-exposed areas. Associated systemic features may occur, but are usually mild. Antibodies to the Ro/SSA antigen are a characteristic finding.

## Antiphospholipid syndrome

This syndrome may be primary (Hughes' syndrome) or occur with SLE. The main features are the occurrence of recurrent miscarriage, venous thromboses, cerebral infarcts, thrombocytopenia and livedo reticularis. These clinical abnormalities are associated with the presence of anticardiolipin antibodies and lupus anticoagulant (subsets of antiphospholipid antibodies).

## Neonatal lupus erythematosus

Neonatal lupus is associated with transplacental passage of maternal anti-Ro and anti-La antibodies. Its features include skin lesions, thrombocytopenia, hepatosplenomegaly and complete heart block. Heart block persists, but the other features resolve as maternal antibodies disappear from the infant's blood.

## Drug-induced systemic lupus erythematosus

Drug-induced SLE is uncommon. The drugs most frequently implicated in its provocation include hydralazine, procainamide, anticonvulsants (phenytoin, primidone), isoniazid and chlorpromazine.

# Dermatomyositis

Heliotrope
*A flower resembling the pale violet,*
*Which, with the Sun, though rooted-fast, doth move*
*And, being changed, yet changeth not her love*
*Ovid*

Dermatomyositis is an autoimmune inflammatory disease of skin and muscle that may occur in childhood or in adult life. There are differences in the manifestations of the disease in these two age groups. Vasculitis and the late development of calcinosis are features of the childhood disease that are not seen in adults. In some adults dermatomyositis is associated with systemic malignancy, whereas there is no association with malignancy in the childhood disease.

## Skin

The skin changes are as shown in the box.

---

**Skin changes**

- Violaceous erythema of the face and V-area of the neck (Figure 17.3). This is said to resemble the colour of the heliotrope flower, and is referred to as 'heliotrope erythema'
- Periorbital oedema
- Erythema on the dorsa of the hands, and linear erythema on the dorsa of the fingers (Figure 17.4). Erythematous papules (Gottron's papules) over the knuckles
- Prominent, ragged cuticles and dilated capillaries in the proximal nail folds (Figure 17.5)
- Erythema over knees and elbows
- In childhood, cutaneous vasculitis leads to ulceration of the skin, particularly in the axillae and groins

Figure 17.3 Facial erythema and periorbital oedema in dermatomyositis.

Figure 17.4 Linear erythema on the dorsa of the hands in dermatomyositis.

3x

Figure 17.5 Hypertrophic cuticle, and nail fold telangiectasia in dermatomyositis.

## Muscles

In some cases there is little evidence of any muscle disease, whereas in others there is profound muscle weakness. Typically, there is symmetrical weakness and wasting of proximal muscle groups, leading to difficulty combing the hair or standing up from a sitting position. Pharyngeal and oesophageal muscles may also be involved, leading to dysphagia.

Other systemic features include interstitial pulmonary fibrosis and cardiac disease (usually manifest as rhythm disturbance or conduction defects).

The reported frequency of malignancy in association with adult dermatomyositis varies widely between series of patients studied, but the incidence seems to be higher in older individuals. The preferred approach to investigation appears to be performance of limited screening, in the form of careful history, thorough physical examination (rectal, lymph node, breast and pelvic examinations), FBC, stool occult blood, cervical smear and chest radiograph. In female patients, ovarian computed tomography (CT) or magnetic resonance imaging (MRI) is advisable. Further investigations should be carried out in anyone with specific symptomatology.

## Investigations

These include skin biopsy, serum levels of muscle enzymes, 24-h urine creatine level, electromyography, muscle biopsy (the triceps muscle preferentially), and ultrasonography and MRI of muscles.

Figure 17.6 A plaque of morphoea.

## Treatment

In dermatomyositis associated with malignancy, there is usually marked improvement when the neoplasm is excised. A relapse of the dermatomyositis signals a recurrence.

The mainstay of therapy is oral corticosteroids. If the response to steroids is poor, immunosuppressives such as azathioprine, methotrexate or cyclophosphamide may be of benefit. Recently, biologic agents have been used with success. Where there is severe muscle involvement, physiotherapy is an important adjunct to drug therapy, in order to minimize contractures.

# Scleroderma

Scleroderma means 'thickening of the skin', and is a term applied to a group of diseases in which there is sclerosis of the skin and destruction of hair follicles and sweat glands. Scleroderma may be an isolated cutaneous phenomenon, when it is called 'morphoea', or a cutaneous component of a multisystem disorder.

## Morphoea

This is a disorder of unknown aetiology in which there is sclerosis of the skin. It may be subdivided clinically into the following types:

1 Circumscribed
2 Linear
3 Frontoparietal (*en coup de sabre*)
4 Generalized

## Circumscribed

This is the most common clinical presentation of morphoea. Solitary or multiple indurated plaques develop, predominantly on the trunk. Initially, affected areas of skin have a violaceous hue, but gradually become thickened and ivory in colour (Figure 17.6). The surface is smooth and shiny. Eventually, usually after many months, the sclerosis resolves, leaving atrophic, hyperpigmented areas.

---

**Classification of scleroderma**

- Morphoea: sclerosis of the skin without systemic involvement
- Systemic sclerosis: cutaneous sclerosis in association with a vasculopathy of small arteries producing multiorgan systemic disease
- Chemically induced scleroderma: sclerosis of the skin as a manifestation of the toxic effects of certain chemicals
- Pseudoscleroderma: sclerosis of the skin associated with a number of diseases other than morphoea or systemic sclerosis

---

## Linear

Linear morphoea usually affects one limb, often extending its full length. In childhood, it can significantly impair the growth of the limb, and produce severe flexion deformities of large joints and digits.

## Frontoparietal (*en coup de sabre*)

Resembling a sabre cut across the scalp and forehead, this type of morphoea is a considerable cosmetic problem. A linear, depressed, sclerotic area extends from the face into the scalp, and is associated with loss of hair along its length.

## Generalized

There is extensive sclerosis of the skin on the trunk and limbs. Flexion contractures restrict limb movement, and if the chest is severely affected breathing may be impaired.

## Treatment

Treatment is often of limited efficacy, but suggested therapies include potent topical steroids, intralesional steroid, topical vitamin D analogues, topical calcineurin inhibitors, UVA and methotrexate. In linear morphoea on the limbs, physiotherapy is essential to maintain joint motility, and orthopaedic surgery may be necessary. Plastic surgery can be of considerable cosmetic benefit in frontoparietal morphoea.

The natural history of morphoea is gradual spontaneous resolution.

# Systemic sclerosis

This is an autoimmune connective tissue disease of unknown aetiology. It is a disorder in which sclerotic changes in the skin occur as one component of a multisystem disorder associated with a vasculopathy of small arteries. In the most common form (sometimes referred to as the CREST syndrome [**c**alcinosis, **R**aynaud's phenomenon, (o)**e**sophageal involvement, **scle**rodactyly and **t**elangiectasia]) skin changes affect predominantly the face and hands.

## Systemic involvement

### Gastrointestinal

Dysphagia is the result of oesophageal involvement. Damage to the myenteric plexus leads to hypomotility of smooth muscle and later to atrophy and fibrosis, resulting in impaired peristalsis. The gastro-oesophageal sphincter mechanism is also impaired, leading to gastro-oesophageal reflux, oesophagitis, and eventual stricture formation. Symptoms of oesophageal reflux are common.

Atrophy and fibrosis of the smooth muscle of the small bowel lead to impaired peristalsis, and the resultant relative stagnation of small bowel contents predisposes to bacterial overgrowth as colonic bacteria move upstream into the small intestine. Gut bacteria deconjugate bile salts (which are essential for micelle formation) and this leads to fat malabsorption and steatorrhoea. Occasionally, patients present with a picture simulating acute intestinal obstruction.

Similar pathology affects the large bowel and leads to the formation of multiple wide-mouthed pseudodiverticula.

### Pulmonary

An inflammatory alveolitis is followed by pulmonary fibrosis, and disease of small pulmonary arteries leads to pulmonary hypertension and cor pulmonale.

---

**Cutaneous features of systemic sclerosis**

**Face**

- The facial skin is sclerotic and bound to underlying structures, producing a tight, shiny appearance, with loss of facial wrinkles, a beaked nose, and restriction of mouth opening (Figure 17.7)
- Perioral furrowing ('purse-string mouth')
- Facial telangiectasia
- Loss of lip vermilion

**Hands**

- Raynaud's phenomenon
- Tight sclerotic skin producing progressive contractures of the digits (sclerodactyly)
- Finger pulp infarcts producing small, painful ulcers (Figure 17.8). These infarctive changes lead to progressive pulp atrophy and resorption of the underlying terminal phalanges
- Calcinosis (Figure 17.9)

---

### Renal

Fibrinoid changes in arteries and arterioles are associated with proteinuria and hypertension. Renal involvement is usually mild, but in some cases it is severe and rapidly progressive, and leads to renal failure.

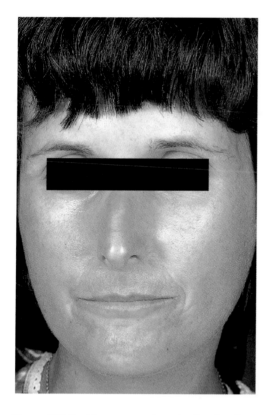

Figure 17.7 Facial appearance in systemic sclerosis.

Figure 17.9 Radiograph showing calcinosis in a digit in systemic sclerosis.

Figure 17.8 Finger pulp ulcers and scars in systemic sclerosis.

## Nervous system

Neurological involvement is uncommon, but carpal tunnel syndrome and trigeminal neuropathy have been reported.

## Cardiac

Myocardial fibrosis, conduction disorders and a variety of ECG abnormalities have been described.

## Hepatic

There is a significant association between systemic sclerosis and primary biliary cirrhosis.

## Musculoskeletal

Arthralgia and arthritis occur in some patients, and myopathy and inflammatory myositis may also occur.

## Treatment

No therapy is known to alter the overall course of systemic sclerosis, but many components of the disease may be helped significantly by specific measures. Digital ischaemia may be helped by electrically heated gloves and socks. Calcium channel blockers may help relieve Raynaud's phenomenon. Patients with oesophageal reflux should avoid lying flat, and treatment with proton pump inhibitors may be very effective. Broad-spectrum antibiotics are helpful in treating patients with gut bacterial overgrowth and malabsorption. The use of angiotensin-converting enzyme (ACE) inhibitors is of significant benefit in renal disease. In interstitial pulmonary disease, cyclophosphamide is effective and bosentan is of benefit for pulmonary arterial hypertension.

## Prognosis

Severe pulmonary or renal involvement is a poor prognostic factor, although treatment is improving, but most patients with systemic sclerosis live for many years.

## Chemically induced scleroderma

Polyvinyl chloride (PVC) can induce a disorder resembling idiopathic systemic sclerosis, and 'vinyl chloride disease' has been described in workers in the PVC industry, particularly reactor cleaners. A number of other chemicals may induce diseases mimicking systemic sclerosis, including perchlorethylene and trichlorethylene (solvents used in dry cleaning), and bleomycin. A disorder similar to systemic sclerosis occurred in 1981 in people poisoned by contaminated rape-seed oil sold as cooking oil in Madrid.

## Pseudoscleroderma

Scleroderma-like changes may be seen in a number of unrelated conditions, including porphyria cutanea tarda, carcinoid syndrome and phenylketonuria.

## Nephrogenic systemic fibrosis

This disorder has been described in recent years and occurs in association with renal insufficiency and exposure to gadolinium-based contrast media. Ill-defined, indurated plaques occur on the trunk and limbs, and histology of these shows thickened collagen bundles, mucin deposition and increased dermal fibroblast-like cells.

# 18

# Pruritus

*There was a young belle of old Natchez*
*Whose garments were always in patches*
*When comment arose*
*On the state of her clothes*
*She drawled: 'When ah itchez, ah scratchez!'*

*Ogden Nash,* Requiem

Pruritus means itching. *Please* note the correct spelling: it is *not* spelt *pruritis*, as often appears in student examination papers, clinical notes and referral letters!

Pruritus varies in duration, localization and severity. Everyone has experienced short-term, localized, itch, and there is a perverse joy in having a really good scratch. However, some individuals have distressing chronic irritation lasting for years. Itching may be restricted to one or more sites, or cover virtually the whole body surface. It may creep about, appearing first on an arm and later on the back, or in more than one site simultaneously. Itching can be mild or appallingly severe, constant and distressing. Chronic pruritus can completely ruin the quality of life.

Pruritus is prominent in many skin diseases. Especially itchy are the eczemas, lichen planus, insect bites and infestations, urticaria and dermatitis herpetiformis. However, the skin may also itch when there is no rash.

The sensation that we call itch is produced, conditioned and appreciated at several levels in the nervous system: stimulus; mediators and receptors; peripheral pathways; central processing; interpretation. A wide variety of stimuli can induce an itch, and a number of chemicals may be involved, especially histamine, prostaglandins and some proteinases. However, the details remain obscure: although histamine can induce itch without producing weals, non-sedative antihistamines have no effect on simple pruritus.

More complex, central mechanisms may also be important in modulating and appreciating pruritus. Many itch-provoking stimuli induce pain if applied at higher intensities. Indeed, scratching appears to induce pain and thereby abolish irritation. However, other sensory stimuli can also overcome itching, and more complex mechanisms have been proposed. One theory involves a complicated filtering system controlling input pathways to further stimuli and passing information on to higher centres.

Itching can certainly be affected by the effects of higher-level brain activity. It is much less apparent when the mind is fully occupied and much worse when boredom sets in. 'Stress' and other psychological factors can induce or worsen pruritus.

## Mechanisms of pruritus

We do not clearly understand why skin diseases itch, and we know very little about irritation in otherwise apparently normal skin.

*Lecture Notes: Dermatology,* 10th edition. © RAC Graham-Brown and DA Burns. Published 2011 by Blackwell Publishing Ltd.

## Causes of pruritus

The term 'pruritus', used without qualification, implies that there is itching without a primary skin disorder. However, in many instances there are considerable secondary skin changes from scratching (e.g. excoriations, scars and prurigo—see below).

But watch out! Subtle changes are easily obscured by scratching: a classic example of this is scabies (see Chapter 5). A full history and a careful examination of the skin are therefore important in all patients complaining of itching.

In considering causes, we look separately at localized itching, generalized states and so-called 'senile' pruritus.

## Localized pruritus

Localized irritation of the skin is common. The skin may be normal, but it is more common to find some abnormalities.

Two very important and troublesome forms of localized pruritus are lichen simplex chronicus and prurigo, and anogenital pruritus.

## Lichen simplex chronicus and prurigo

This difficult problem is sometimes called 'neuro-dermatitis'. It is thought that constant irritation leads to constant scratching which, in turn, leads to thickening of the skin. This may occur in plaques, known as lichen simplex chronicus (Figure 18.1), or in nodules, which are given the name prurigo (Figure 18.2). The areas are intensely irritable, and a self-perpetuating itch–scratch cycle develops. Patients who develop this kind of localized itching are often rather tense.

### Sites of predilection

Classic sites for lichen simplex chronicus include the shins, forearms, palms and back of the neck (sometimes known as 'lichen nuchae'); perianal and vulval skin may also be affected (see below). Prurigo nodules may accompany areas of lichen simplex or appear separately almost anywhere; they are frequently multiple.

Lesions are often asymmetrical.

Figure 18.1 Lichen simplex chronicus.

Figure 18.2 Nodular prurigo.

## Treatment

Potent topical steroids (sometimes under occlusive bandages) may help, but the problem often recurs.

## Anogenital pruritus

Two very common (and least talked about) forms of localized itching are pruritus vulvae and pruritus ani. They may be encountered together.

Pruritus ani is often attributed to haemorrhoids. However, although haemorrhoids and tags are often present, their treatment alone does not always relieve the symptoms. The problem is also often dismissed as psychological, but only rarely is this the complete explanation.

Anal itching may continue for years. Irritation is often spasmodic and extremely intense. Most patients are male.

### Clinical features

Examination often reveals little abnormality; there may be some excoriation and thickening of anal and perianal skin; 'tags' are often present; occasionally gross changes amounting to lichen simplex are seen, when the charming term 'mossy bank anus' may be applied; there may be an associated fissure.

### Aetiology

Pruritus ani is probably largely a low-grade irritant reaction to faeces, sweat and discharge; sedentary occupations make matters worse. Contact allergy to medicaments may be a factor, especially allergy to local anaesthetics and preservatives. Psoriasis of the natal cleft and perineum may give rise to pruritus ani.

Pruritus vulvae can be very distressing. There are a number of causes to consider (see Table).

## Generalized pruritus

Persistent generalized pruritus is extremely unpleasant, and can either affect most of the body surface continuously or involve several different areas. By definition, a primary skin disorder has been excluded.

### Clinical features

Skin changes vary considerably—nothing to see at all; mild flakiness of the skin, with a few scratch marks; or the skin may be covered in excoriations,

---

**Causes of pruritus vulvae**

- Mild incontinence (with prolapse) may cause irritant changes
- Skin disorders: notably eczema, psoriasis and lichen sclerosus (et atrophicus) (see Chapter 15)
- Allergic contact dermatitis to medicaments (as in anal itch—see above)
- Candidiasis (secondary to diabetes): the vulva is beefy red, and there may be pustules and a vaginal discharge
- Vulval itch with no visible signs, when a true psychogenic origin is suspected

---

**Treatment of perineal irritation**

This depends upon the cause.

*'Irritant' pruritus ani*
- Good hygiene, a high-fibre diet and treatment with topical steroids are useful
- Treating concomitant haemorrhoids may reduce discharge

*Skin disorder and allergic contact dermatitis*
- Most will require topical steroids

*Candidiasis*
- Antifungal creams and pessaries; check for diabetes

*No changes seen*
- Patients seldom respond to antipruritics
- Inexpert psychological probing is valueless

---

scars and nodules. The skin is often dry, especially in elderly patients.

Although there may be no identifiable underlying disorder, all patients with generalized irritation should be investigated because a number of potentially remediable systemic disorders may be responsible.

## Haematological disorders

Chronic iron deficiency may be due to blood loss (e.g. from menorrhagia or a gut carcinoma). Many elderly patients and some vegans are iron deficient for dietary reasons. Polycythaemia rubra vera is characteristically associated with itching triggered by bathing.

## Systemic disorders causing irritation

**Haematological disorders**
- Iron deficiency
- Polycythaemia rubra vera

**Cholestatic liver disease**
- Extrahepatic obstruction
- Primary biliary cirrhosis
- Hepatitis
- Drug-induced cholestasis

**Chronic renal failure**

**Thyroid disease**
- Thyrotoxicosis
- Myxoedema

**Malignancy**
- Lymphomas and leukaemias
- Carcinomas

**Drug ingestion**
- Especially opiates

**Pregnancy (see Chapter 15)**

Up to 30% of Hodgkin's disease patients have generalized pruritus.

## Drugs

Various agents induce itching, but the mechanisms are poorly understood. Opiates appear to act centrally and on mast cells. Oestrogens and phenothiazines induce cholestasis.

## Diabetes mellitus

You may come across lists quoting diabetes as a cause of itching, but we do not consider that this is the case.

## Psychological factors

When everything else has been excluded, psychological factors may be considered. The most common underlying problem is an anxiety neurosis, but patients with monodelusional psychoses such as parasitophobia also itch. These individuals, however, offer their own explanation only too readily! (see Chapter 20).

Screening procedures for generalized pruritus are as shown in the box.

## Liver disease

The itch is probably related to bile salts in the skin. Irritation may precede the development of other features of cholestatic liver disease, especially in primary biliary cirrhosis.

## Chronic renal failure

Unfortunately the intractable itch of renal failure is largely unaffected by dialysis. Parathyroidectomy is said to help, but the benefit is short-lived and is hardly justified in most patients.

## Thyroid disease

Both thyrotoxicosis and myxoedema may present with pruritus. In myxoedema the general dryness of the skin may be responsible.

## Cancers

Lymphoreticular malignancies are particularly prone to cause itching, but pruritus may also occur in association with a variety of carcinomas.

## Screening for generalized pruritus

- A full history and general examination
- Full blood count
- Erythrocyte sedimentation rate (or plasma viscosity)
- Liver function tests
- Blood urea/urea nitrogen/creatinine
- Iron studies
- Serum thyroxine
- Urine protein
- Chest radiograph

If these tests are negative initially and, if the pruritus persists, repeat at intervals

## Treatment

Treatment of generalized pruritus is that of its cause. When no apparent underlying reason can be found, a topical steroid and a sedative antihistamine, such as hydroxyzine, may help. Some authorities recommend opiate antagonists. UVB phototherapy may help, as may gabapentin.

## 'Senile' pruritus

Itching with no apparent cause is common in elderly people. It may be mild and localized, but can be very severe and generalized. The patients (and their carers) are often anxious and miserable, but this is usually secondary to the irritation rather than a primary cause. This state is called 'senile pruritus'. It is not known what causes ageing skin to itch.

## Examination

The skin is texturally either 'normal' or 'dry'. Excoriations, secondary eczematization and areas of infection are common. Localized areas of 'eczema craquelé' may develop (see Chapter 7).

## Treatment

Treatment is extremely difficult. Sedative antihistamines often cause excessive drowsiness and confusion, and topical steroids are of limited use. If the skin is texturally 'dry', liberal use of emollients may be helpful. Care has to be taken, however, as these agents can make both the patient and their surroundings very slippery!

Increased frequency of washing or the use of harsh soaps and detergents makes matters worse, both by removing surface lipids and by acting as direct irritants. Soaps should therefore be used sparingly and emollients employed instead.

# 19

# Systemic disease and the skin

The skin may be involved directly or indirectly in a number of systemic disease processes, and can provide visible diagnostic clues that could lead to the discovery of internal disease.

## Endocrine disease

### Diabetes

There are a number of cutaneous manifestations of diabetes, including those in the box.

> **Cutaneous features**
>
> 1 Certain cutaneous infections
> 2 Neuropathic ulcers
> 3 Necrobiosis lipoidica
> 4 Diabetic dermopathy
> 5 Diabetic bullae
> 6 Xanthomas
> 7 Acanthosis nigricans
> 8 Lipoatrophy
> 9 Cheiroarthropathy

*Lecture Notes: Dermatology*, 10th edition. © RAC Graham-Brown and DA Burns. Published 2011 by Blackwell Publishing Ltd.

1 Cutaneous infection: mucosal candidiasis, particularly balanoposthitis and vulvovaginitis, and carbuncles, occur more frequently in people with diabetes
2 Neuropathic ulcers: impaired sensation, as a result of sensory neuropathy, predisposes to the development of neuropathic ulcers on the soles of the feet (Figure 19.1)
3 Necrobiosis lipoidica: lesions of necrobiosis lipoidica characteristically occur on the shins, although they may develop elsewhere. The lesions are initially erythematous, but subsequently become yellowish-brown and atrophic, and underlying blood vessels are easily seen through the thinned skin (Figure 19.2). Occasionally the lesions ulcerate. Good diabetic control does not appear to influence the skin lesions. Potent topical steroids and intralesional steroid injections are among several treatments suggested for necrobiosis lipoidica, but results of therapy are not very impressive
4 Diabetic dermopathy: this term is applied to small, brown, scar-like lesions seen on the shins in some people with diabetes. The lesions are thought to be associated with diabetic microangiopathy
5 Diabetic bullae: in this uncommon blistering disorder of people with diabetes, subepidermal bullae occur on the hands and feet. Their aetiology is unknown

Figure 19.1 Diabetic neuropathic ulcer.

Figure 19.2 Necrobiosis lipoidica with a small ulcerated area.

6 Xanthomas: hyperlipidaemia in uncontrolled diabetes may be associated with the development of multiple small, yellow, eruptive xanthomas

7 Acanthosis nigricans: in association with insulin resistance

8 Lipoatrophy: insulin-resistant diabetes associated with partial or generalized cutaneous lipoatrophy

9 Cheiroarthropathy: a scleroderma-like thickening of the skin of the hands in people with type 1 diabetes

## Granuloma annulare

There is no significant association between classic granuloma annulare and diabetes, but in a much rarer generalized form of granuloma annulare there is an association with diabetes. Typically, lesions of granuloma annulare are groups of firm, skin-coloured papules, often arranged in rings, and commonly occurring on the dorsa of the hands and feet (Figure 19.3). The natural history of granuloma annulare is eventual spontaneous resolution, but persistent lesions may be treated with intralesional triamcinolone or cryotherapy.

# Thyroid disease

## Hypothyroidism

The skin is typically dry, and feels thickened due to subcutaneous mucin deposition—hence the designation myxoedema. A malar flush on an otherwise pale face produces what has been referred to as a 'strawberries and cream' appearance. There may be a yellowish tinge to the skin, said to be due to the deposition of carotenes. There is often periorbital oedema. Scalp hair is diffusely thinned and there is loss of the outer part of the eyebrows. Sitting close to the fire to keep warm may produce severe erythema ab igne ('granny's

Figure 19.3 Granuloma annulare.

tartan') on the shins, but since the advent of central heating this physical sign has become uncommon.

## Hyperthyroidism

Cutaneous changes that may accompany thyrotoxicosis include excessive sweating, palmar erythema, diffuse alopecia, generalized hyperpigmentation and thyrotoxic acropachy (digital clubbing). The nails may show onycholysis. Some patients develop pretibial myxoedema, which is produced by subcutaneous deposition of excessive amounts of mucopolysaccharide, and is characterized by erythema and thickening of the soft tissues over the shins and dorsa of the feet.

Vitiligo may accompany autoimmune thyroid disease, and generalized pruritus may be a feature of both hypo- and hyperthyroidism.

## Adrenal disease

### Cushing's syndrome

The cutaneous effects of Cushing's syndrome include thinning of the skin, spontaneous bruising, prominent striae on the trunk and limbs, diffuse alopecia, acne and hirsutism.

### Addison's disease

Diffuse hyperpigmentation is the main cutaneous manifestation of Addison's disease. The pigmentation is particularly prominent on the buccal mucosa and in the palmar creases. Vitiligo may also accompany autoimmune Addison's disease.

## Rheumatic diseases

### Gout

In addition to tophaceous deposits around affected joints, gouty tophi may occur on the ears.

### Still's disease

This is a disorder of childhood, although it may rarely occur in adults. Accompanying the pyrexial episodes of Still's disease is a diffuse maculopapular eruption that characteristically develops in the late afternoon and evening, and usually resolves by the following morning. Some slander-mongers claim that dermatologists never see this eruption because its periodicity is outside their normal working day!

### Rheumatoid arthritis

Dermatological features of rheumatoid arthritis include those in the box.

**Dermatological features**

- Rheumatoid nodules: subcutaneous nodules over bony prominences, particularly on the extensor aspect of the forearms and the dorsa of the hands
- Vasculitic lesions: digital vasculitis may produce small infarcts around the nail folds (Bywaters' lesions), or more severe digital ulceration and even gangrene. Vasculitic lesions may also occur on the legs, and contribute to the development of leg ulcers
- Pyoderma gangrenosum
- Palmar erythema

## Rheumatic fever

Almost extinct in developed countries, rheumatic fever may be accompanied by a characteristic eruption, erythema marginatum.

## Reiter's disease (reactive arthritis)

Predominantly a disease of young adult males, Reiter's disease is a reactive arthropathy usually precipitated by non-specific urethritis, but occasionally by bacillary dysentery. In addition to urethritis, conjunctivitis/uveitis and arthritis, there may be an eruption that is indistinguishable from psoriasis. On the soles of the feet the skin lesions may become extremely thickened, producing so-called 'keratoderma blenorrhagicum'. The buccal mucosa may show scattered erosions, and superficial circumferential erosive changes on the penis are referred to as 'circinate balanitis'.

# Vitamin deficiency

## Scurvy

The classic picture of vitamin C (ascorbic acid) deficiency is rarely seen nowadays in developed countries, but scurvy may be encountered in elderly people and in people with alcohol problems, as a result of nutritional self-neglect. The typical appearance is of perifollicular purpura, easy bruising, poor wound healing and bleeding gums.

## Pellagra

Pellagra is the result of nicotinic acid deficiency. Classically, it has three major manifestations—dermatitis, diarrhoea and dementia. The dermatitis affects light-exposed areas, and there is often a well-demarcated margin to the affected area on the neck (Casal's necklace). Pellagra may occur in people with alcohol problems as a result of nutritional self-neglect, and in food faddists. A similar dermatitis may be provoked by isoniazid in individuals who are slow acetylators of this drug.

# Inflammatory bowel disease

Ulcerative colitis and Crohn's disease may be associated with a number of mucocutaneous manifestations including those in the box.

**Mucocutaneous features**

- Pyoderma gangrenosum: the lesions may be single or multiple. They initially resemble boils, which subsequently break down to form necrotic ulcers with undermined purple edges (Figure 19.4). Pyoderma gangrenosum may also occur in association with rheumatoid arthritis, myeloma and leukaemia. The treatment of choice is systemic steroids, but a variety of other treatments including azathioprine, minocycline, clofazimine and ciclosporin may also be effective
- Erythema nodosum
- Perianal and buccal mucosal lesions: in Crohn's disease, anal examination may reveal fleshy tags, fissures and perianal fistulae. The buccal mucosa may be oedematous and ulcerated, and the lips may be swollen as a result of a granulomatous cheilitis

# Hyperlipidaemia

Both primary and secondary hyperlipidaemic states may be associated with lipid deposits in the skin, known as xanthomas. There are several different clinical types of xanthomas. Orange–yellow

Figure 19.4 Pyoderma gangrenosum.

Figure 19.5 Xanthelasma.

in association with tendons, often involving the Achilles tendons and extensor tendons on the dorsa of the hands. Deposits of lipid in the skin creases of the palms of the hands (striate palmar xanthomas; Figure 19.7) appear to be particularly associated with primary type III hyperlipidae-mia (broad beta disease; dysbetalipoproteinae-mia). Eruptive xanthomas are crops of yellowish papules that occur in association with marked hypertriglyceridaemia.

# Amyloidosis

In systemic amyloidosis, amyloid deposits in the tongue produce macroglossia, and cutaneous deposits are visible as yellowish, waxy, purpuric plaques around the eyes and in the perianal area.

lipid deposits in the eyelid skin are known as xan-thelasma (Figure 19.5). Tuberous xanthomas occur as yellowish nodules, usually over bony prominences (Figure 19.6). Tendinous xantho-mas, as their name suggests, are deposits of lipid

Figure 19.6 Tuberous xanthomas.

Figure 19.7 Striate palmar xanthomas.

# Sarcoidosis

Sarcoidosis is a multisystem granulomatous disorder of unknown aetiology. There are a number of patterns of skin involvement in sarcoidosis, including those shown in the box.

> **Skin patterns**
>
> - Erythema nodosum: tender, erythematous nodules on the legs (see Chapter 16)
> - Lupus pernio: the skin of the nose and ears is involved in the granulomatous process, and becomes swollen and purplish in colour
> - Scar sarcoid: sarcoid granulomas localize in old scar tissue, making the scars prominent
> - Papules, nodules and plaques: these often have an orange–brown colour

# Liver disease and the skin

Changes in the skin and nails that occur in association with chronic liver disease include those in the box.

> **Skin and nail changes**
>
> - Palmar erythema
> - Pruritus: in cholestatic liver disease
> - Spider naevi: in a superior vena caval distribution
> - Xanthelasma: in primary biliary cirrhosis
> - White nails (Terry's nails)
> - Pigmentary changes: in addition to jaundice, patients with longstanding cholestatic liver disease may also have marked melanin pigmentation; patients with haemochromatosis have generalized bronze-brown pigmentation that is produced by a combination of iron and melanin

# Cutaneous manifestations of systemic malignancy

## Cutaneous metastases

Malignant tumours may metastasize to the skin, and tumours of renal, ovarian, gastrointestinal, breast and bronchial origin are those most likely to do so. Cutaneous metastases usually present as pink nodules, and occur most frequently on the scalp and anterior trunk. Scalp metastases may produce areas of alopecia (alopecia neoplastica).

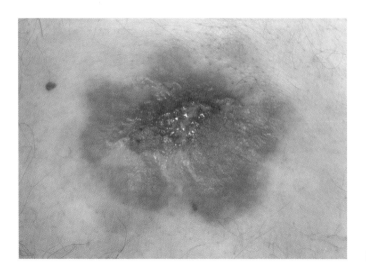

Figure 19.8 Sister Joseph's nodule.

Lymphatic extension of carcinoma to the skin may produce an area of erythematous induration resembling cellulitis, and known as 'carcinoma erysipeloides'.

Metastasis of ovarian or gastrointestinal carcinoma via the ligamentum teres can present as an umbilical nodule (Sister Joseph's nodule; Figure 19.8).

## Miscellaneous cutaneous signs of underlying malignancy

1 Dermatomyositis (see Chapter 17)
2 Acanthosis nigricans: this is a warty, hyperpigmented thickening of skin in the flexures (Figure 19.9). The palms of the hands may also be affected, producing an appearance known as 'tripe palms'. The most common associated malignancy is an adenocarcinoma of the gastrointestinal tract. However, 'malignant' acanthosis nigricans is rare
3 Generalized pruritus: generalized itching, without a rash, may be associated with a wide variety of systemic malignancies
4 Thrombophlebitis migrans: this is particularly associated with carcinoma of the pancreas
5 Acquired ichthyosis: ichthyosis developing for the first time in adult life may be associated with a lymphoma
6 Pyoderma gangrenosum: this may occur with myeloma and leukaemia
7 Necrolytic migratory erythema: this is a distinctive eruption associated with pancreatic glucagonoma

Figure 19.9 Acanthosis nigricans.

8 Flushing and a rosacea-like eruption are cutaneous features of the carcinoid syndrome
9 Erythema gyratum repens: this rare skin marker of malignancy is a bizarre eruption with an appearance resembling wood grain
10 Acquired hypertrichosis lanuginosa: the sudden growth of profuse vellus hair over the face and body is a rare sign of underlying neoplastic disease
11 Paraneoplastic pemphigus: this rare blistering disorder typically occurs in patients with lymphoproliferative diseases

# Leukaemia and the skin

There are numerous cutaneous changes that may accompany leukaemia, or be provoked by the drugs used in its treatment.

Common presenting features of acute leukaemia include purpura, bruising and bleeding from the gums, and the skin may be directly involved in the form of leukaemic infiltrates. Disseminated herpes zoster (herpes zoster with numerous outlying vesicles) may accompany leukaemia, as may a severe bullous form of pyoderma gangrenosum, and Sweet's disease (acute febrile neutrophilic dermatosis).

# Purpura

Purpura is produced by extravasation of red cells into the skin, and has numerous causes. The lesions do not blanch on pressure.

Causes of purpura include vasculitis (see Chapter 16), quantitative or qualitative platelet abnormalities, drugs, amyloidosis, dysproteinaemias and infections (e.g. meningococcaemia).

# AIDS and the skin

Patients with the acquired immunodeficiency syndrome (AIDS) are at increased risk of developing a number of mucocutaneous problems:

1 Oral candidiasis extending into the oesophagus
2 Oral 'hairy leukoplakia': white ridges along the sides of the tongue, caused by the Epstein–Barr virus
3 Seborrhoeic dermatitis: this is often severe, and is probably related to an altered host response to malassezia yeasts
4 Papular pruritic eruption and eosinophilic folliculitis are manifest as itchy papular lesions and are signs of advanced immunosuppression. They are probably part of the same spectrum. Their aetiology is unknown
5 Staphylococcal infection, shingles, molluscum contagiosum and dermatophyte fungal infection occur more commonly in AIDS patients
6 Episodes of herpes simplex are more frequent and more severe, and lesions may become chronic
7 Perianal warts tend to be more florid and more difficult to treat
8 Kaposi's sarcoma: a tumour that is thought to arise from vascular endothelium and is related to infection with human herpesvirus type 8 (HHV-8). Lesions are usually multiple, and may affect any part of the skin, as well as internal organs. It is rarely the cause of death in AIDS patients, who usually succumb to intercurrent infection. It is a radiosensitive tumour
9 Pre-existing psoriasis may become severe and extensive in AIDS patients
10 Bacillary angiomatosis: caused by the bacillus *Bartonella henselae*, these angioma-like lesions affect the skin, mucosae and internal organs. They respond to treatment with erythromycin
11 Drug-associated problems: the antiretroviral treatment now widely employed in treating HIV infection may provoke rashes and cause nail pigmentation. In addition, a cosmetically troublesome lipodystrophy, characterized by symmetrical loss of subcutaneous fat, that on the face produces a cachectic appearance, is associated with highly active antiretroviral therapy (HAART)

# 20

# Skin and the psyche

*If you happen to have a wart on your nose or forehead, you cannot help imagining that no one in the world has anything else to do but stare at your wart, laugh at it, and condemn you for it, even though you have discovered America.*

*Fyodor Dostoevsky*, The Idiot

Patients with skin disease who often ask 'Is it caused by nerves doctor?' are usually trying to establish if they can attribute their skin condition to 'stress'. In fact, few skin disorders are directly related to psychological disturbance. However, there is evidence that psoriasis and atopic eczema may be exacerbated by stress, and other conditions in which emotional stress has been claimed to play a part in some cases include alopecia areata and acute pompholyx.

There is no doubt that skin disease has psychological effects on the patient, and can significantly adversely affect their quality of life. Skin disease is visible to others, it carries the taint of contagion, and affected individuals often feel stigmatized and have poor self-image and low self-esteem. They will be aware that their skin is being scrutinized, and that any form of physical contact, such as shaking hands or collecting change, may provoke apprehension in others. In certain ethnic groups where marriages are arranged, the presence of skin disease may compromise marriage prospects, and cause considerable emotional distress.

Infections with ectoparasites sometimes have marked psychological effects. Patients feel unclean, and these feelings can persist long after the problem has been eradicated.

*Lecture Notes: Dermatology*, 10th edition. © RAC Graham-Brown and DA Burns. Published 2011 by Blackwell Publishing Ltd.

There are some skin disorders that are directly related to psychological problems, and these are described below.

## Dermatitis artefacta

Patients with dermatitis artefacta produce skin lesions to satisfy a psychological need, but what benefit they derive from their actions is usually not obvious. There is no rational motive for their behaviour. They will vehemently deny that the lesions are self-induced if challenged. As a group they are distinct from malingerers, who consciously imitate or produce an illness for a deliberate end.

Dermatitis artefacta is more common in women, and most of those affected are adolescents or young adults. However, there is a subgroup with an older age of onset who are more likely to be male. Many have some connection with the health professions, either directly or via family members.

Artefactual skin lesions may be produced in a number of different ways including rubbing, scratching, picking, gouging, puncturing, cutting, sucking, biting, the application of heat or caustics, or the injection of milk, blood and faecal material. Limb oedema may be simulated by the intermittent application of constricting bands (Secretan's syndrome). Lesions tend to have bizarre geometric shapes that do not conform to those seen in naturally occurring disease—no dermatosis has square, rectangular or triangular lesions. Often the lesions are more numerous on the side of the body opposite the dominant hand. If a caustic material such as an acid has been used to induce lesions this may trickle off the main area of damage to produce the 'drip-sign' of tell-tale streaks at the margins. Even when suspected artefactual lesions are covered with occlusive dressings, patients will often manage to insert knitting needles under the dressings, or push sharp instruments through them, in order to continue damaging the skin.

The history obtained from these patients is devoid of any useful information about the evolution of their lesions. The impression conveyed is that one minute the skin was normal, and the next it was blemished. This so-called 'hollow history' is characteristic, as is a striking complacency about what are often extremely disfiguring lesions ('*la belle indifference*'), sometimes accompanied by an enigmatic 'Mona Lisa' smile. One patient we have seen, who had extensive suppuration of the left arm, probably produced by the inoculation of faeces (Figure 20.1), said about her arm 'Yes, it is rather unpleasant isn't it. I wonder if you could arrange for someone to take it off'.

When they see the severity of the lesions and an apparent lack of progress in diagnosis and treatment, relatives and friends of the patient quite naturally rally to their support, and may be somewhat vocal in their criticism of a seemingly inept medical profession. Other doctors caring for the patient may also be convinced that their disease is naturally occurring. This situation, in which other individuals 'support' a patient with dermatitis artefacta, is known as '*folie à deux*', and is also encountered in delusions of parasitosis (see below).

The psychopathology of patients who produce artefactual lesions is not uniform, but in some cases there is a demonstrable personality disorder, and in others significant depression.

It requires considerable expertise to be able to make a confident diagnosis of dermatitis artefacta, but even experienced dermatologists see cases in which they suspect the lesions are self-induced, but they cannot be certain. Alternatively, there are occasional cases in which there is a strong suspicion of dermatitis artefacta, but the lesions are discovered to be the result of naturally occurring disease.

Treatment is extremely difficult in many cases. Confronting the patient with the diagnosis achieves very little, in that it usually produces a categorical denial that they are producing the lesions, and subsequent failure to attend for follow-up. Strict occlusion of the traumatized areas may allow healing, but the lesions will reappear as soon as occlusive dressings are removed. An alarming consequence of occlusion may be the appearance of lesions elsewhere, or the development of other 'symptoms', as if to compensate for the inability to reach the usual sites. Antidepressants will help those who are depressed. Psychiatric referral is often unhelpful and, unfortunately, many patients refuse assistance from a psychiatrist. The situation often remains at a stalemate. As long as the doctor's suspicions are not voiced, the patient appears content to continue attending for follow-up.

The course of this disorder is often protracted. Recovery often has little to do with successful medical treatment, but occurs because of increasing maturity, marriage or having children. However, there are some physicians who have

Figure 20.1 Dermatitis artefacta—in this case probably the result of inoculation of faeces into the skin.

expertise in psychocutaneous disorders, and referral to such a specialist is advisable.

# Dermatological pathomimicry

Dermatological pathomimicry is distinct from dermatitis artefacta. Patients with this condition either deliberately perpetuate their skin disease, or reproduce a pre-existing skin disorder. Having been appraised of the aetiology of their skin disease, they use this knowledge to reproduce the lesions when under emotional stress, to obtain sympathy, or in an effort to avoid an unpleasant situation with which they cannot cope. Examples of the type of illness used by patients for pathomimicry include allergic contact dermatitis, drug reactions and chronic leg ulceration.

Sympathetic discussion with the patient will usually solve the problem.

# Body dysmorphic disorder (dermatological non-disease; dysmorphophobia)

In this condition patients complain of severe symptomatology localized to certain parts of the body, most commonly the face, scalp and perineum, but without any objective evidence of disease. The complaints include: dysaesthesias such as burning, itching or throbbing pain; too much or too little hair on the face or scalp, or altered texture of scalp hair. Perineal symptoms in men include complaints of a red, burning scrotum. These delusional beliefs or perceptions of abnormal sensations are a consuming preoccupation for the patient. There is nothing abnormal to see on examination, but the perceived abnormalities often lead to consultations for 'remedial' cosmetic surgery, and most are dissatisfied with the results of this.

In some cases depression is part of the picture; others may be have monosymptomatic hypochondriacal psychosis. There is a significant risk of suicide. Management is difficult, but some patients respond to treatment with antidepressants and cognitive–behavioural therapy.

# Delusions of parasitosis

The individual with delusions of parasitosis has an unshakeable conviction that his or her skin is infested with parasites. An experienced dermatologist will recognize this disorder from information supplied in the referral letter, and will often arrange to see the patient at the end of a clinic, because the consultation is usually extremely lengthy. However, before seeing a dermatologist the patient has often consulted his or her local university department of zoology or a medical entomologist in an attempt to identify the 'parasites'. They will also probably be known to companies specializing in pest eradication, who will have been asked to disinfest their home. They may have isolated themselves from family and friends because of their fear of passing the 'infestation' on to them, and because of their absolute conviction that they are infected they may have convinced their family, friends, and even the family doctor, of the reality of the problem (shared delusion; *folie à deux*).

Patients often describe a feeling of itching, biting or 'crawling' in the skin (formication), and state that when this occurs they are able to remove a small 'insect' or 'worm' from a skin 'lesion'. When asked to demonstrate typical skin 'lesions', they will often point to Campbell de Morgan spots, freckles or other minor blemishes. Typical 'specimens' are presented to the doctor wrapped in pieces of paper or adhesive tape, and kept in a matchbox (Figure 20.2). These should always be

Figure 20.2 Matchbox and 'specimens' in delusions of parasitosis.

Figure 20.3 Trichotillomania.

examined under the microscope, because they just might contain parasites, but usually they contain fragments of cotton or skin debris.

It is impossible to persuade these patients that parasites are not responsible for their condition. If they are shown that their 'specimens' are simple debris they remain unconvinced, and may even suggest that the parasites are so small that an electron microscope will be required to demonstrate them. In this situation the most lucid, eloquent discourse will fall upon deaf ears—the patient's beliefs remain unshaken, and the doctor usually retires from the conflict feeling more than somewhat jaded.

Delusions of parasitosis has been described in association with a number of medical disorders, including organic brain disease such as senile dementia and cerebral arteriosclerosis, pellagra, vitamin $B_{12}$ deficiency and after coronary bypass surgery. The term 'monosymptomatic hypochondriacal psychosis' may be applied to patients with a single, fixed delusion, and most patients with delusions of parasitosis fit into this category.

Effective treatment is very difficult, and many patients continue with their delusion for years. As with dermatitis artefacta, a confrontational approach rarely achieves anything. Patients often refuse psychiatric help because they do not accept that they have a mental illness, and cannot see how a psychiatrist could possibly help with what, to them, is a physical disorder. The neuroleptic drug pimozide was employed in the past, but it is now considered that newer antipsychotic agents such as risperidone and olanzapine are preferable. As with other psychocutaneous disorders, physicians with a special interest in the condition should be consulted.

# Obsessive–compulsive habits

## Trichotillomania

Trichotillomania means compulsive plucking of hair. The scalp is involved most often, but the eyebrows and eyelashes may be affected. A mild form of trichotillomania may be observed in libraries, where engrossed students compulsively twist locks of hair around their fingers, but they rarely pull it out unless examinations are approaching! The clinical picture is of patches of hair loss containing hairs of varying length. Often the crown of the head is affected, and the hair at the margins is of normal length (Figure 20.3). The underlying scalp is usually normal, but may be excoriated. Occasionally, trichotillomania is associated with a trichobezoar (hair ball in the stomach) if the plucked hair is swallowed. 'Rapunzel's syndrome' (named after the character in the Grimm Brothers' fairy tale) is applied to individuals in whom the hair forms a tail extending into the small intestine.

Trichotillomania in childhood is often transient. However, it may be a manifestation of significant psychopathology, particularly in adults.

## Pathological skin picking

'Neurotic excoriations' is a term for a disorder, encountered predominantly in middle-aged women, in which skin lesions are produced by picking and gouging, and are usually scattered over the arms, upper trunk and face. More recent lesions are usually interspersed with scars from previous excoriations. Acne excoriée is a variant of this condition in which minimal acne lesions are repeatedly picked and gouged, leaving scars when the lesions heal.

Patients with these problems have obsessive–compulsive personalities, and picking the skin appears to provide relief of unconscious aggression and tension. Antidepressants and supportive psychotherapy may be of benefit.

# 21

# Cutaneous drug reactions

*There are only two types of drug—those that don't work and those that have side-effects.*

Bruno Handel FRCS

## Introduction

The skin is one of the most common sites for unwanted drug effects (a better term than 'side effects'), although estimates of the frequency vary considerably. Cutaneous drug reactions are probably under-reported and certainly often go unrecognized. Note, however, that skin disorders wholly unrelated to drug ingestion can be labelled erroneously. It is important not to jump to conclusions: we have seen viral infections and scabies diagnosed as drug reactions. There are many people who state that they are 'allergic to penicillin', but who are not.

Cutaneous drug reactions may be due to several different mechanisms. Unfortunately there are no reliable in vitro tests for establishing that a rash is due to a drug. Simple in vivo tests, such as prick testing and patch testing, have a limited place in specific situations, but usually yield no useful information either. However, even if the mechanism(s) for a particular reaction is known (and it often isn't), a test may not be appropriate because the reaction is not to the drug itself, but to a drug complex or metabolite that is produced in vivo after ingestion or administration.

The only definitive test is direct challenge with the suspected agent, but this may be impossible or unethical in many circumstances. For these reasons, proving that a specific eruption was due

to a specific drug is difficult, and judgements usually have to be made on clinical grounds alone.

---

**Causes of drug reactions**

- Simple intolerance
- Hypersensitivity: types I, II, III and IV
- Pharmacokinetic disturbances
- Drug interactions
- Complex interactions between host, drug and environment (e.g. light)

---

## Drug reaction patterns

However, all is not lost! Some drugs are much more prone to induce cutaneous drug reaction patterns than others. Common offenders include those in the box.

---

**Drugs causing skin reactions**

- Antibiotics (especially penicillin, semisynthetic penicillins and sulfonamides)
- Non-steroidal anti-inflammatory drugs
- Hypnotics
- Tranquillizers

---

Furthermore, there are a number of well-defined clinical drug reaction patterns. Some of these patterns are more specific to certain drugs, and this may help to identify the culprit.

*Lecture Notes: Dermatology*, 10th edition. © RAC Graham-Brown and DA Burns. Published 2011 by Blackwell Publishing Ltd.

> **Common cutaneous drug reaction patterns**
>
> - Exanthematic eruptions
> - Urticaria and anaphylaxis
> - Exfoliative dermatitis
> - Vasculitis
> - Fixed drug eruptions
> - Lichen planus-like eruptions
> - Erythema multiforme
> - Acneiform eruptions
> - Hair abnormalities
> - Pigmentary changes
> - Bullous reactions
> - Photosensitivity
> - Lupus erythematosus-like syndrome
> - Exacerbation of pre-existing skin disease

## Exanthematic eruptions

The most common cutaneous drug reactions are itchy, widespread, symmetrical, erythematous and maculopapular (Figure 21.1): there is often a strong resemblance to a viral exanthem. The time relationship is variable: in most instances the rash begins a few days after starting the drug, but it may begin almost immediately, or be delayed for a few weeks. Exanthematic eruptions usually fade a week or so after stopping the drug, but exfoliative dermatitis may develop (see below and Chapter 15).

### Common causes

Non-steroidal anti-inflammatory drugs and antibiotics, particularly ampicillin, other semisynthetic penicillins, sulfonamides and gentamicin.

### Rarer causes

Gold, barbiturates and phenothiazines.

## Urticaria and anaphylaxis (see also Chapter 15)

Drug-induced urticaria may be due to a direct pharmacological action on mast cells, or to type I or type III hypersensitivity reactions.

Occasionally, drugs may trigger a major anaphylactic reaction, with or without urticaria, which can be fatal unless treated very rapidly. Unfortunately, there is no way of predicting this disaster.

### Common causes

Aspirin, opiates (direct), penicillins, cephalosporins, pollen vaccines and toxoids (immune).

## Eczema

Type IV hypersensitivity reactions to topical medicaments are common, and give rise to a contact dermatitis (see Chapter 7). Figure 21.2 shows a man who was given eyedrops containing neomycin (an aminoglycoside). Occasionally, a topically sensitized patient may receive the compound (or a closely related chemical) systemically. The result is a severe, widespread, eczematous reaction.

### Common causes

Lanolin in creams and bandages; preservatives (parabens, ethylenediamine) in creams; topical anaesthetics (*not* lidocaine); topical antihistamines; topical antibiotics, especially aminoglycosides, in creams and drops; increasingly, topical steroids.

## Exfoliative dermatitis

Drugs are one of the four important causes of exfoliative dermatitis (see Chapter 15).

### Common causes

Prominent offenders are sulfonamides and sulfonylureas, gold, phenytoin, allopurinol and barbiturates.

## Vasculitis (see Chapter 16)

Drug ingestion is a common trigger for vasculitis.

### Common causes

Thiazides, captopril, cimetidine, quinidine, sulfonamides.

## Fixed drug eruptions

Fixed drug eruptions are one of the most curious events encountered in dermatological practice. The reaction occurs in the same place(s) every time the offending drug is taken. They are often misdiagnosed as recurrent eczema or ringworm.

A round or oval patch of dusky erythema develops, often with a purplish centre (Figure 21.3), and sometimes a central bulla. This fades to leave postinflammatory hyperpigmentation. There may be only one lesion or multiple sites. Fixed erup-

Figure 21.1 A typical exanthematic eruption due to an antibiotic.

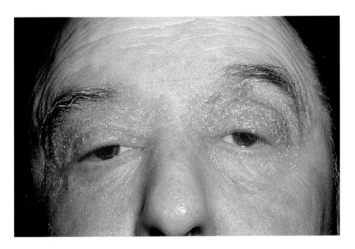

Figure 21.2 Contact sensitivity to neomycin.

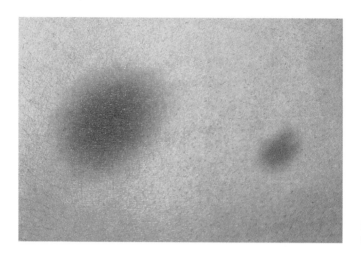

Figure 21.3 Fixed drug reaction to a sulfonamide.

tions can occur anywhere, but the limbs and genitalia are favoured sites.

### Common causes

Sulfonamides, dapsone, tetracyclines, barbiturates.

## Lichen planus-like eruptions

Lichen planus-like (sometimes known as 'lichenoid') reactions are rare, but can be severe. The eruption is occasionally indistinguishable from idiopathic lichen planus, but more commonly there is an eczematous element, with much more scaling. In severe cases, an exfoliative dermatitis may develop (see above and Chapter 15).

### Causes

Antimalarial drugs; some β blockers; sulfonylureas; gold. Thiazides may cause lichen planus-like eruptions on light-exposed surfaces.

## Erythema multiforme (see Chapter 15)

So many things seem to be able to trigger erythema multiforme that it is usually difficult to be certain whether a drug is responsible.

### Suggested drug causes

Barbiturates; long-acting sulfonamides; co-trimoxazole; rifampicin.

## Acneiform eruptions

Skin changes resembling acne vulgaris occur with several drugs. The changes tend to be monomorphic, consisting largely of papulopustules. There are seldom comedones present.

### Causes

Corticosteroids (both topical and systemic), adrenocorticotrophic hormone (ACTH), androgenic drugs, lithium and iodides. Some drugs also exacerbate pre-existing acne (see below).

## Hair abnormalities

As discussed in Chapter 13, drugs may be responsible for hair loss or excessive hair growth.

## Pigmentary changes

Several drugs cause pigmentary changes (Table 21.1).

Heavy metals such as silver may be deposited in the skin after industrial exposure or ingestion (e.g. in antismoking lozenges).

## Bullous reactions

There are several ways in which drugs may induce blistering.

## Drug-induced blistering

- In fixed drug eruptions
- Drugs may induce pemphigus and pemphigoid (see Chapter 14)
- Drugs may exacerbate porphyria cutanea tarda
- Nalidixic acid may cause a dramatic phototoxic bullous reaction
- Barbiturates may be associated with bullae on bony prominences, usually in patients who are unconscious due to overdose

**Table 21.1 Drugs causing cutaneous pigmentary changes**

| Colour | Drug |
| --- | --- |
| Characteristic generalized reddish-brown hue | Clofazimine (used in leprosy) |
| Yellow | Mepacrine |
| | Carotene |
| Purplish | Chlorpromazine |
| Blue–black | Chloroquine (especially on shins) |
| | Minocycline (in high dosage) |
| | Amiodarone (on light-exposed sites) |
| Brown | Oestrogens (=chloasma) |

# Photosensitivity

There are three main types of reaction (see box).

## Photosensitive reactions

- Exacerbation of underlying disease
- Direct phototoxic reaction
- Photoallergic reaction

In phototoxic reactions, the dose of the drug and the intensity of ultraviolet exposure may both be important: if critical levels are not reached, the reaction may not develop. This can be confusing if the drug has been taken on a number of occasions.

Figure 21.4 Photosensitivity to a sulfonamide.

Patients complain that exposure to the sun causes a burning sensation followed by erythema, swelling and, later, eczematous changes on light-exposed areas (Figure 21.4).

## Common causes

Phenothiazines; sulfonamides; tetracyclines; thiazides. Demethylchlortetracycline can cause photo-onycholysis. Bullae due to nalidixic acid have been mentioned above.

# Lupus erythematosus-like syndrome

A rare but important drug reaction is the induction of a syndrome closely resembling systemic lupus erythematosus.

## Causes

Many agents have been incriminated, including hydralazine, isoniazid, penicillin, minocycline, procainamide and griseofulvin.

## Exacerbation of pre-existing disease

Some drugs may produce a deterioration in certain skin disorders. Notable examples are:

1 Acne: androgenic drugs (e.g. danazol, stanozolol), oral contraceptives and corticosteroids
2 Porphyrias: all clinical features, including cutaneous photosensitivity, may be worsened by drug ingestion, particularly barbiturates and oestrogens
3 Psoriasis: lithium, antimalarials
4 Systemic lupus erythematosus: penicillin and sulfonamides may produce deterioration

### Clinical information

- A good history
- A careful examination
- Elimination of other skin diseases
- Recognition of the clinical reaction pattern
- Matching the reaction with the most likely offender
- Tests, where appropriate (possibly including a challenge)

# Conclusion

If you use all the clinical information at your disposal, it is often possible to determine if a rash is drug provoked, and what the causative agent might be.

# 22

# Treatment of skin disease

*If it's dry, wet it. If it's wet, dry it. Congratulations, you are now a dermatologist!*

Anonymous

The above witticism is oft quoted by non-dermatologists as an assessment of the scope of dermatological therapeutics. An alternative calumny relates to a dermatologist murmuring an unintelligible Latin name as a diagnosis and then prescribing a topical steroid, for everything. Apart from being deeply offensive to sensitive skin doctors, both these quips are far from the truth, as dermatologists have an enormous therapeutic armamentarium at their disposal. In days of yore, it must be admitted, many of the available topical therapies resembled witches' brews containing 'Eye of newt and toe of frog, wool of bat and tongue of dog'. They were often cosmetically unacceptable and malodorous—if the skin disease did not render the patient a social pariah, the treatment could be relied upon to do so. However, in recent years, topical therapies have not only become more effective, but also cosmetically much more acceptable.

The treatment of individual disorders has been dealt with in preceding chapters, and this chapter is designed to provide an overview of the principles of therapy.

## Topical therapy

With regard to topical therapy, an ideal preparation for the management of skin disease would

*Lecture Notes: Dermatology*, 10th edition. © RAC Graham-Brown and DA Burns. Published 2011 by Blackwell Publishing Ltd.

penetrate well, but remain localized within the skin, thereby avoiding potential problems from systemic effects. In practice this is extremely difficult to achieve, and any agent that penetrates the stratum corneum is absorbed to some extent.

Topical preparations consist of an active ingredient (or ingredients) and a material in which this is suspended—a base. These components must be compatible. There is little point in discovering a new base that penetrates the skin like a hot knife through butter if it completely inactivates everything suspended in it.

The stratum corneum forms a natural protective barrier to penetration of externally applied agents. Hence, to facilitate penetration by a drug, this barrier function must be breached, and this can be achieved by hydration of the stratum corneum, e.g. penetration of a topical steroid may be markedly enhanced by occluding an area of skin with polythene. Unfortunately, if large areas of skin are occluded in this way the amount of steroid absorbed may be sufficient to produce systemic effects. Bases containing urea also hydrate the stratum corneum and enhance penetration of their active ingredients. Dimethyl sulfoxide (DMSO) is a solvent that penetrates skin extremely rapidly, and is used as a vehicle for the antiviral agent idoxuridine.

## Bases

Bases include creams, oily creams, ointments, lotions, gels and pastes. A cream is an oil-in-water emulsion that is relatively non-greasy and has only limited emollient activity. Creams are cosmetically acceptable and can be used to treat either moist or dry skin conditions. Oily creams are water-in-oil emulsions that combine good emollient properties with cosmetic acceptability and are therefore of benefit in dry skin conditions. Ointments are greasy preparations that have emollient and occlusive properties. The occlusive effect of an ointment results in hydration of the stratum corneum and enhanced penetration of the active ingredient of the ointment. The benefits of ointments are offset by a lack of cosmetic acceptability. Ointments are messy and stick to clothing. If used on the hands they transfer to everything touched—an obvious disadvantage to someone employed in clerical work, for example. Lotions are fluid preparations that have a cooling effect due to evaporation. They are useful in the management of moist, exudative skin lesions, and also in dermatoses affecting the scalp. Clear, non-greasy gels are designed for use on hairy parts of the body, where they are cosmetically acceptable. Pastes are powders, usually mixed with soft paraffin, and are protective, e.g. in the prevention of maceration of the skin around a discharging ulcer.

The choice of a particular base should be determined by the type of skin problem and the sites affected. It is, for example, wholly inappropriate to prescribe a steroid ointment for daytime use on the scalp, because it is too messy. A gel or lotion preparation should be used instead. Similarly, a lotion is not the correct base for ichthyotic skin, where an oily cream or ointment is more appropriate.

Bases are mixtures of several components, formulated to provide stability and freedom from microbial contamination. Random dilution of a topical preparation will dilute the preservatives in the base and significantly shorten its shelf-life.

# Communication and patient compliance (adherence)

Most non-topical medication involves popping pills of various colours into the mouth at certain times of the day, requiring a minimum of effort and only a minor feat of memory. Topical therapy demands a great deal more of the patient, and the increased effort required of the patient ought to be matched by the provision of precise instructions by the doctor. Verbal instructions are not sufficient if multiple topical therapies are prescribed. For example, a patient with psoriasis might be given a tar shampoo, a steroid scalp lotion, a mild topical steroid cream to use in the flexures, and a vitamin D analogue for plaques on the trunk and limbs. If the patient has only recently developed psoriasis, and is not familiar with its treatment, the provision of multiple therapies without clear instructions could easily lead to confusion.

Do not expect patients who depart for work at the crack of dawn to adhere strictly to instructions to wash their hair every morning and use a topical medication twice daily. Modify the treatment schedule to suit the individual. If you are prescribing a preparation that is messy to use and/or malodorous, warn the patient about this, e.g. dithranol stains and benzoyl peroxide bleaches, and lack of prior warning could lead to ruined clothing and bedsheets.

It is a useful exercise to imagine how strictly you would adhere to a regimen if you were encumbered with a skin disease requiring regular treatment.

# Quantities prescribed

It is important when prescribing topical therapy to consider the area to be covered and the frequency of application before assessing the quantity of a topical agent required by the patient, e.g.

**Table 22.1 Steroid potency**

| Potency | Examples |
| --- | --- |
| Mild | 0.1–2.5% hydrocortisone |
| Moderately potent | Clobetasone butyrate (Eumovate) |
| | Fludroxycortide (Haelan) |
| | Alclometasone dipropionate (Modrasone) |
| | Hydrocortisone with urea (Alphaderm) |
| Potent | Betamethasone valerate (Betnovate) |
| | Fluocinolone acetonide (Synalar) |
| | Fluocinonide (Metosyn) |
| | Hydrocortisone butyrate (Locoid) |
| Very potent | Clobetasol propionate (Dermovate) |
| | Diflucortolone valerate (Nerisone Forte) |

there is little point in prescribing a 30-g tube of an emollient to be used over the entire body surface after bathing—this hardly constitutes a week's supply for an ichthyotic gerbil. A repeat prescription would be required after one application, because this is the approximate amount necessary for a single application over the whole body surface of an adult. Topical therapies are available in a variety of container sizes. You will need to check the available sizes before prescribing, as they vary from product to product. Topical steroids, for example, may be marketed in 15-, 25-, 30-, 50- or 100-g tubes, depending on the manufacturer and the steroid. Most emollients are available in 50- and 100-g tubes and 500-g tubs or dispensers.

Underprescribing and overprescribing are both common. One does not require 100 g of cream to treat a small patch of eczema on the leg—most of the tube will languish in a drawer or bathroom cabinet until its shelf-life is long expired, or it may be inappropriately used by another member of the family. However, someone regularly using an emollient over extensive areas of skin should be given 500-g dispensers.

# Topical steroids

At first sight the huge number of available topical steroids is bewildering to the uninitiated, but with a little knowledge and experience their use is quite straightforward. They are divided into several groups according to potency. Hydrocortisone preparations are the weakest. However, hydrocortisone in a base containing urea, which enhances penetration of the stratum corneum, is moderately potent. Modification of the basic steroid skeleton by fluorination (fluorinated steroids) or esterification produces steroids of much greater potency (Table 22.1).

## Choice of preparation

The most appropriate topical steroid for a given situation should be determined by the type and severity of the condition being treated, the sites affected and the age of the patient. The skin disorders that are steroid responsive have been delineated in previous chapters, and include various types of eczema, lichen planus, psoriasis of the scalp, flexures, hands and feet, and discoid lupus

erythematosus. In general, a severe dermatosis should be treated with a potent steroid, and a mild condition with a weak steroid. In the case of a chronic dermatosis subject to periodic exacerbations a mild-to-moderate potency steroid can be used when the condition is quiescent, and a potent preparation when it worsens.

There are regional variations in the absorption of topical steroids through the skin and their potential for local adverse effects. These variations are determined by the thickness of the stratum corneum, occlusion, e.g. in the flexures where skin surfaces are in apposition, and the vascularity of the area. Most facial dermatoses should be treated only with mild topical steroids, although a few conditions such as discoid lupus erythematosus will require potent preparations. Skin disease affecting the axillae, groins and submammary areas should also be treated with mild topical steroids. Conversely, dermatoses of the palms and soles, where the stratum corneum is extremely thick, require potent steroids, and a greater benefit is often obtained if polythene occlusion is used to enhance penetration.

There is a greater risk of adverse systemic effects from the use of topical steroids in children because of the high ratio of skin surface area to body volume, particularly in infants. For this reason mild topical steroids should be used in small children. The skin of elderly people is thin, and potent steroids will amplify this change—their use over long periods of time should therefore be avoided or carefully supervised.

## Side effects

Side effects are rarely seen after the use of mild topical steroids, but they are encountered more frequently in association with potent topical steroid use, although much less commonly than in the early years of steroid availability.

Side effects may be divided into local, occurring at the site of application of the steroid, and systemic, resulting from percutaneous absorption.

### Local side effects

#### Atrophy of the skin

Topical steroids produce dose-related thinning of the dermis as a result of inhibition of fibroblast activity. This effect is particularly noticeable in areas where the skin is naturally relatively thin, such as the axillae, medial aspect of the upper arm, groins and the medial aspect of the thigh. Prominent striae may develop in these areas (Figure 22.1). On the face, cutaneous thinning and telangiectasia produce prominent erythema. Frequent use of potent steroids on the dorsa of the hands and the forearms results in easy bruising, particularly in elderly people (Figure 22.2).

## Hypopigmentation

Inhibition of melanocyte function leads to hypopigmentation. In parts of the world where potent topical steroids are readily available without prescription, they are sometimes used for their skin lightening action, leading to other damaging effects. Local loss of pigmentation in racially pigmented skin is sometimes seen after steroid injections.

## Perioral dermatitis

Perioral dermatitis is a condition usually seen in young women who have used potent topical steroids on the face for lengthy periods of time—often inappropriately for mild acne on the chin. The eruption consists of small papules and pustules on an erythematous background (Figure 22.3). The history is virtually identical in all cases. Initially the mild acne appears to improve, probably because the vasoconstrictor action of the steroid reduces erythema, and inflammatory papules become less noticeable. However, stopping treatment results in a rebound flare of the erythema, and the patient therefore considers that the treatment is keeping the condition controlled and continues to apply the steroid; she may even increase the frequency of application. Eventually,

Figure 22.1 Prominent striae in the axilla after use of a potent topical steroid.

as the eruption around her mouth becomes more noticeable, she asks her doctor for 'something stronger', and is often given a more potent topical steroid.

Figure 22.2 Severe atrophy of skin on the dorsa of the hands after excessive use of fluorinated topical steroids.

Figure 22.3 Perioral dermatitis.

Treatment consists of explaining the nature of the condition, stopping the potent topical steroid, warning the patient about the rebound flare of erythema, and prescribing a mild topical steroid (1% hydrocortisone) for 2–3 weeks to reduce its severity. In addition, oxytetracycline or erythromycin should be given in a dose of 500 mg twice daily, gradually reducing over a period of several weeks as the condition improves. The reason for their efficacy is unknown.

### Steroid rosacea

Topical steroids will worsen pre-existing rosacea, and can precipitate a rosacea-like eruption.

### Allergic contact dermatitis

Allergic contact dermatitis to topical steroids may develop, usually in patients using them long term, e.g. in the treatment of atopic dermatitis (see Chapter 7).

### Pustular psoriasis

If large quantities of a potent topical steroid are used inappropriately to treat psoriasis, and the treatment is then suddenly stopped, the psoriasis may exacerbate dramatically and pustular psoriasis may occur.

### Infection

Folliculitis may occur in areas treated with topical steroids, particularly when ointments or polythene occlusion are used, and the use of steroids on moist, warm flexural areas may encourage superinfection with *Candida* spp. Inappropriate use of topical steroids on dermatophyte fungal infections alters the appearance of the eruption, producing so-called 'tinea incognito' (see Chapter 4). Scabies inappropriately treated with topical steroids becomes extremely florid, with many burrows and a very numerous mite population (see Chapter 5).

## Systemic side effects

Topical steroids are absorbed through the skin, and excessive use of potent steroids may result in inhibition of the pituitary–adrenal axis and iatrogenic Cushing's syndrome. This problem is rarely encountered nowadays, because doctors are aware of the adverse effects, and restrict the amounts prescribed. In children, growth retardation is an important consequence of the long-term use of potent topical steroids.

## Topical immunomodulators

In recent years the immunomodulators (calcineurin inhibitors) tacrolimus and pimecrolimus, the mechanism of action of which is similar to that of ciclosporin, but which penetrate the stratum corneum more readily because they have a lower molecular weight, have emerged as useful topical agents. They are licensed for use in atopic eczema, but may also be of benefit in other conditions, including discoid lupus erythematosus, vitiligo and alopecia areata, and to date they appear to have a good safety profile.

## Vitamin D analogues

Principally used in the topical treatment of plaque psoriasis, vitamin D analogues are of benefit because of their potent antiproliferative effect and ability to promote normal differentiation. Preparations containing calcipotriol, calcitriol and tacalcitol are marketed for psoriasis treatment, but have been used with benefit in a number of other disorders. Recently, a combination of calcipotriol and betamethasone dipropionate has been marketed.

Use of excessive amounts of these products leads to hypercalcaemia and hypercalciuria, and it is therefore important to follow prescribing guidelines.

## Retinoids

### Retinoic acid (tretinoin)

This is used in the treatment of acne (see Chapter 6). It is particularly effective in reducing the number of comedones. It is also used in the management of photoageing and, usually in combination with other agents, to reduce hyperpigmentation, e.g. in chloasma.

### Adapalene

This is a synthetic retinoid that is used in the treatment of acne.

### Tazarotene

This is also a synthetic retinoid, which is used in the treatment of acne and psoriasis.

# Systemic therapy

## Retinoids

### Isotretinoin (13-*cis*-retinoic acid)

The introduction of this drug transformed the management of severe acne, and in recent years many dermatologists have used it for less severe acne unresponsive to other forms of treatment. The usual treatment regimen is 0.5–1.0 mg/kg body weight per day for 16–24 weeks, which produces prolonged remission in many patients. If the acne becomes troublesome again, or is unresponsive to the first course, then treatment may be repeated. The principal effect of the drug is a reduction in the size of sebaceous glands and reduced sebum production. This is accompanied by a secondary reduction in the bacterial flora of the pilosebaceous follicle.

Potential adverse effects include dryness of the lips, nasal mucosae (with mild epistaxes) and conjunctivae, decreased night vision, diffuse thinning of hair, myalgia and arthralgia, benign intracranial hypertension (avoid concomitant tetracyclines) and hyperlipidaemia. Mood changes may occur in patients taking isotretinoin, but whether there is a direct relationship between the drug and depression is a controversial issue. However, if depression is identified the drug should be stopped.

Isotretinoin is a teratogen, and sexually active women of child-bearing age should take strict contraceptive precautions for at least 1 month before, during, and for at least 1 month after treatment— guidelines with regard to pregnancy testing and contraception are available.

## Acitretin

This is the active metabolite of etretinate. It is useful in extensive psoriasis and pustular psoriasis (but less so in stable plaque psoriasis), and in the ichthyoses and Darier's disease. Acitretin is also of value in tumour prevention in individuals predisposed to skin neoplasia such as those with xeroderma pigmentosum and post-transplantation patients on long-term immunosuppression.

Potential adverse effects are similar to those associated with isotretinoin. However, with regard to teratogenicity, as there is reverse metabolism of acitretin to etretinate, and the latter has a long elimination half-life, women of child-bearing age should use contraceptive precautions for the duration of treatment and for at least 2 years after stopping the drug.

## Alitretinoin (9-*cis*-retinoic acid)

This has recently been introduced for the management of patients with severe chronic hand eczema. Adverse effects are similar to those from other oral retinoids, and a pregnancy prevention programme is mandatory in women of child-bearing age.

## Methotrexate

A structural analogue of folic acid, methotrexate is a competitive inhibitor of the enzyme dihydrofolate reductase that converts dihydrofolate to tetrahydrofolate, the latter being important in the synthesis of RNA/DNA. It is used in the treatment of severe psoriasis and psoriatic arthritis, where its benefit is thought to depend on inhibition of pro-liferation of lymphoid cells. It may also be of benefit in other diseases, including sarcoidosis, lupus erythematosus and dermatomyositis.

It is usually given orally as a single weekly dose (7.5–15 mg weekly; with lower doses in elderly people). Concomitant folic acid administration is recommended (1–5 mg daily), as this protects against some of the adverse effects without affect-ing response to therapy.

Major adverse effects are pancytopenia and hepatotoxicity (fibrosis and cirrhosis). Factors predisposing to the latter include excessive alcohol intake and viral hepatitis.

Certain drugs elevate methotrexate levels and therefore increase the risk of toxicity, and these include NSAIDs, trimethoprim and sulfamethoxazole.

Monitoring of treatment should include initial frequent measurement of full blood count and long-term assessment of a serological marker of fibrosis, PIIINP (the amino-terminal peptide of type III procollagen). If levels of PIIINP remain normal there is unlikely to be liver damage, but if levels are repeatedly raised then further assess-ment by liver biopsy is indicated.

## Azathioprine

Azathioprine is converted in the body to 6-mercaptopurine, an immunosuppressive agent. It may be of benefit in several disorders, including dermatomyositis, systemic lupus erythematosus, immunobullous diseases and vasculitis. Dosage is 1–3 mg/kg per day. Major adverse effects include hypersensitivity reactions, bone marrow suppres-sion and hepatotoxicity.

Important in the catabolism of azathioprine is the enzyme thiopurine methyltransferase (TPMT), and some individuals have genetically determined low activity of this enzyme, rendering them par-ticularly susceptible to myelosuppression. Anyone considered for azathioprine therapy should have blood TPMT levels measured.

## Ciclosporin

Ciclosporin, a calcineurin inhibitor, is a potent immunosuppressant. In dermatology it is princi-pally used in treating severe psoriasis and atopic dermatitis, but its other uses include pemphigus and pemphigoid, dermatomyositis and pyoderma gangrenosum.

Its main adverse effects are hypertension and nephrotoxicity. It interacts with numerous other drugs. Monitoring of therapy should include reg-ular measurement of blood pressure and serum creatinine.

## Biologic interventions

A major development in therapeutics in recent years has been the introduction of 'biologic thera-pies', a group of agents that block specific molecu-lar steps in the inflammatory process. Their principal dermatological use is in the manage-ment of moderate-to-severe psoriasis, when tradi-tional systemic treatments have failed or are contraindicated. The agents currently employed are tumour necrosis factor (TNF) antagonists (inf-liximab, adalimumab and etanercept) and they are administered intravenously (infliximab) or subcutaneously (adalimumab and etanercept). TNF is a proinflammatory cytokine that plays a central role in the pathogenesis of psoriasis. Biologic therapies may have significant adverse effects, and it is essential that treatment guide-lines be strictly followed. They are expensive.

# 23

# Emergency dermatology

## Introduction

Dermatological emergencies are rare, but early recognition and referral are just as important in dermatology as in any other branch of medicine. You are most likely to pick up the specifics of management if you encounter one of these situations while in your first years in medicine.

## Toxic epidermal necrolysis and Stevens–Johnson syndrome (see Chapters 14 and 15)

Although technically these are separate conditions, we are considering them together for the purposes of this discussion. They are blistering diseases that occur secondary to cutaneous inflammation, where the inflammation of the epidermis results in very serious damage. The changes may be so severe that the epidermal layer dies and is shed, leaving an exposed, oozing dermis. In general, Stevens–Johnson syndrome is restricted to mucous membranes with a mild bullous disorder on the skin, whereas in toxic epidermal necrolysis (TEN) most of the skin is involved (see Figure 14.12). The skin can initially become itchy or patients may complain of a burning sensation and a fever. Mucosal involvement is common and internal epithelial surfaces

*Lecture Notes: Dermatology*, 10th edition. © RAC Graham-Brown and DA Burns. Published 2011 by Blackwell Publishing Ltd.

(gastrointestinal tract, lung, etc.) may also be involved. Early referral either to specialist centres with highly experienced dermatology nursing care and a general intensive care unit (ICU) or a burns unit gives patients the best chance of survival. Beyond general measures there is some debate as to best treatment, but intravenous immunoglobulin and ciclosporin can be given as additional measures.

## Erythroderma (see Chapter 15)

If you have read the previous chapters in this textbook, you will know that erythroderma is not a pathological diagnosis. However, there are only a few conditions that commonly cause this state to develop, and identification of the cause is essential to successful management. The term essentially refers to the clinical state of inflammation of all the skin. Given that the skin is the largest organ of the body, it is not surprising that this can result in haemodynamic and metabolic problems:

- Hypothermia from heat loss
- High-output cardiac failure
- Hypoalbuminaemia
- Fluid loss
- Capillary leak syndrome: a very severe complication, where cytokines released during inflammation cause generalized vascular leakage; it most commonly occurs in erythroderma secondary to psoriasis; acute respiratory distress syndrome can result, and this invariably requires ICU management

The four most important causes of erythroderma are:

1 Dermatitis (eczema), including contact allergic
2 Psoriasis
3 Cutaneous T-cell lymphoma
4 Drugs (stopping all non-essential drugs is often a good idea)

Involving dermatological services in an attempt to establish the most likely cause and to advise on specific management is often necessary. However, general treatment measures should be instituted immediately (Table 23.1).

# Meningococcal septicaemia

Meningococci can cause the most severe forms of progressive meningitis and 'sepsis syndrome'. The latter syndrome may result in disseminated intravascular coagulation, which gives the characteristic rash that the general public associates with 'meningitis', but importantly occurs only when the inciting pathogen is a meningococcus. The classic description is of a purpuric rash that spreads rapidly and does not blanch when pressure is applied (note in the earliest stages the rash can blanch). Any patient with such a rash requires

---

### Table 23.1 Treatment measures for erythroderma

**General**

Keep the patient warm

Swab the skin for secondary bacterial infection

Monitor vital signs

Monitor serum albumin

Keep meticulous fluid balance charts

**Specific**

Simple emollients and mild topical steroids

The blanket use of systemic steroids should be avoided in the absence of high-output cardiac failure: they can complicate further management of disease and there are obvious side-effects associated with their use

Treatment as for the underlying cause (e.g. methotrexate for psoriasis)

A similar approach should be taken in the treatment of pustular psoriasis (see Chapter 8).

---

urgent investigation and the involvement of senior colleagues. Note, too, that a strong clinical suspicion of bacterial meningitis is one situation where immediate treatment of disease takes precedence over investigations. Immediate intravenous antibiotics may be life saving.

---

# Necrotizing fasciitis

This is an extremely dangerous condition, which can be very difficult to diagnose, as very little can sometimes be seen from a surface inspection. There are two forms of the condition: type 1 is caused by aerobic and anaerobic bacteria and is often seen postoperatively; type 2 is caused by a group A streptococcus and can arise spontaneously in healthy individuals. In both cases the infection spreads beyond the subcutis into underlying fascia and muscle: this is deeper than simple cellulitis infection and, contrary to popular belief, the two are not a continuum. Clinically affected areas become disproportionately painful compared with other clinical signs. Necrosis is rapid and can result in septicaemia and death. If there is even the slightest suspicion of necrotizing fasciitis, the involvement of senior colleagues and urgent surgical intervention are essential. Intravenous antibiotics used alone are ineffective because the blood supply is compromised and vessels cannot deliver antibiotics to the necrotic tissues in sufficient concentration. Surgical debridement (which sometimes means amputation of part/all of a limb) is always indicated, combined with postoperative high-dose intravenous antibiotics.

---

# Kaposi's varicelliform eruption (disseminated herpes simplex/eczema herpeticum)

This can be a very severe disease and is seen in patients who have large areas of broken skin. The most common condition that predisposes to disseminated herpes simplex is atopic eczema, but it can also be associated with other dermatoses such as pemphigus foliaceus or Darier's disease (a relatively common genodermatosis—see Chapters 3, 11 and 14). A typical history consists of preceding malaise and fever in a patient known to have atopic dermatitis, followed by a widespread vesicular rash that quickly breaks down to leave eroded areas. Patients can become systemically unwell and a small number of cases develop a viraemia and/or meningoencephalitis. Management is hospital based and involves general supportive measures, such as intravenous fluids and antipyretics, but definitive treatment is with intravenous antiviral therapy in the toxic patient (it is reasonable to use oral aciclovir in the afebrile patient). Also remember to stop any non-essential therapies, including topical steroids. It is common practice to give broad-spectrum antibiotic cover to stop superimposed bacterial infection. Crucially, if there is any evidence of ocular involvement, early ophthalmological review is essential.

# Angioedema (and anaphylaxis)

Angioedema is usually a type 1 hypersensitivity reaction characterized by swelling of the dermis, subcutaneous tissues and mucosae. Triggers can be allergic or non-allergic, but the final pathway in both cases is the release of inflammatory mediators, such as histamine, from mast cells, causing fluid to leak from blood vessels and resulting in tissue swelling. A similar process occurs in urticaria, but here only superficial vessels in the upper dermis are affected. The same picture can also result from non-IgE mediated reactions, (e.g. to aspirin and non-steroidal anti-inflammatory drugs [NSAIDs]), and non-allergic mechanisms (e.g. to angiotensin-converting enzyme [ACE] inhibitors) where the chemical responsible is bradykinin not histamine.

The key issue in managing a patient with angioedema is assessing the airway and ensuring that it remains patent. It is important to remember that 'anaphylaxis' can present with life-threatening **a**irway and/or **b**reathing and/or **c**irculation (ABC) problems and should consequently be dealt with via the method of assessment and treatment, as taught in the Advanced Life Support Guidelines (ALS ) by the Resuscitation Council (UK). It must also be pointed out that skin and mucosal changes are subtle/absent in 20% of reactions.

Management should follow the ALS guidelines, and involves high-flow oxygen, an initial dose of 0.5 mg intramuscular adrenaline at a concentra-

**Table 23.2 Management of severe angioedema and anaphylaxis**

Oxygen

0.5 mg intramuscular 1 : 1000 adrenaline

Intravenous antihistamine

Intravenous corticosteroid

Intravenous infusion

tion of 1 : 1000 (note that the concentration in cardiac arrest is 1 : 10000 administered intravenously), and intravenous fluid if hypotensive (Table 23.2). Antihistamines (e.g. chlorphenamine 10 mg i.m./i.v.) and corticosteroids should also be administered for allergic-type reactions. Most importantly, given the life-threatening nature of angioedema and anaphylaxis, while carrying out your initial assessment and management it is imperative to contact senior doctors (including an anaesthetist) so that they are aware of the problem, and will be able to help, especially if initial management is unsuccessful.

# Staphylococcal scalded skin syndrome (SSSS)

Whereas staphylococcal skin infections are commonplace, fortunately 'staphylococcal scalded skin syndrome' is extremely rare. It is a blistering disorder caused by exfoliative toxins that are produced by some types of staphylococci, and cause the skin to peel away, leaving a scalded/burned appearance. Treatment is with intravenous antibiotics and general supportive measures such as intravenous fluids and good nursing and nutritional care.

# Final word

Dermatological emergencies need early identification and prompt management by experts, and nobody will expect junior doctors to manage these complicated conditions on their own. However, basic knowledge of these disorders will enable them to initiate swift and appropriate action, because it is speed of intervention that proves life saving in most cases.

# Case study questions

## Case study 1

A 75-year-old woman has had scaly patches below the knees for several years. They were thought to be plaques of psoriasis, but standard topical therapies for psoriasis have been ineffective. Recently, a fleshy tumour has developed on one of the scaly areas.

**Examination**
There are several pink, scaly patches on both legs below the knee (Figures C1.1 and C1.2), and a tumour on the left calf (Figure C1.3). There are a few solar keratoses on the face and dorsa of the hands, but the rest of the skin is normal. The nails are normal.

What are the scaly patches, and what is the tumour?

Figure C1.1

Figure C1.2

Figure C1.3

## Case study 2

A fit, 4-year-old child has two asymptomatic lesions on the dorsum of the left foot that have been present for 6 months and have not responded to topical antifungal agents.

**Examination**
There are two annular lesions on the dorsum of the foot (Figure C2.1). The slightly raised margin of each lesion is composed of pink papules. There is no scaling.

What is the diagnosis?

Figure C2.1

## Case study 3

An 18-year-old woman, an apprentice hairdresser with a past history of childhood eczema and asthma, presents with an itchy rash on both hands. She has been working in a hairdressing salon for several months, and spends most of her time shampooing clients' hair.

**Examination**

There is diffuse redness and scaling of the dorsa of the hands (Figure C3.1).

What are the possible causes, and what investigations should be performed?

Figure C3.1

## Case study 4

What is the likely diagnosis in each of these patients who have rashes affecting the feet?

(a) A scaly, non-itchy eruption (Figure C4.1) accompanied by similar lesions on the knees, elbows and scalp, and a nail dystrophy.

(b) An intensely itchy, weeping rash on both feet (Figure C4.2).

(c) An itchy, dull red rash on both feet, with a scaling margin (Figure C4.3). The patient also recently developed an itchy rash in the groins.

Figure C4.1

Figure C4.2

Figure C4.3

## Case study 5

A 90-year-old woman has a lesion on the nose. It has been present for several years, during which time it has slowly enlarged.

**Examination**

There is a flat, heavily pigmented area on the nasal bridge (Figure C5.1).

What is the diagnosis, and what treatment would you suggest?

Figure C5.1

## Case study 6

A child, who has had an itchy flexural rash for several years, has developed multiple small spots scattered over the body, but they are more numerous in areas affected by the pre-existing dermatosis. Both of the child's siblings have similar lesions.

### Examination

There are a large number of pink papules, each of which appears to have a central plug, and some of which are inflamed (Figure C6.1). The elbow and knee flexures are red, scaly and moist (Figure C6.2).

What are the papular lesions, and what is the background dermatosis?

Figure C6.1

(a)

Figure C6.2

(b)

## Case study 7

This man complained of an itchy rash on the beard area that had been present for several weeks. It had not been treated.

**Examination**

There is redness and scaling affecting the left side of the jaw and extending onto the neck. The involved area has a distinct, scaly erythematous margin (Figure C7.1).

What is the diagnosis?

Figure C7.1

## Case study 8

A 65-year-old woman, who had complained of itching for several weeks with little to see, has suddenly developed crops of blisters.

**Examination**

There are extensive areas of tense bullae, some of which are haemorrhagic (Figure C8.1). Her mouth is not involved.

What is the likely diagnosis?

Figure C8.1

## Case study 9

A 30-year-old man, a keen squash player, has had an itchy rash in the groin for several months. Topical therapy with several steroid preparations has produced some reduction in the intensity of itch, but the rash has gradually become more extensive. On further questioning he admits to a problem on his feet for years.

### Examination

There is patchy scaling erythema on the medial aspects of the thighs, and numerous inflammatory papules and pustules (Figure C9.1).

What is the diagnosis?

## Case study 10

A 40-year-old patient was started on an ACE inhibitor for elevated blood pressure. Three weeks later the patient awoke in the middle of the night with swollen lips and eyes.

What is the most likely diagnosis? What action would you take?

Figure C9.1

## Case study 11

A 75-year-old former sailor complains of a lesion on the back that
he has noticed because it has
bled and marked his shirts.

### Examination
Overlying the right shoulder
there is a raised lesion that has an
eroded central area (Figure C11.1
(a) & (b)), the source of the bleeding, but there is also a pigmented
lesion in the centre of the back, of
which the patient had not been
aware. The latter is an irregular
area of dark pigmentation with
an adjacent small erosion (Figure
C11.1 (c)).

What are the lesions most likely
to be?

Figure C11.1

## Case study 12

A 21-year-old university student has had dandruff and a scaly scalp since his early teens. In the past 3 weeks he has developed a widespread eruption of lesions on the trunk. These were preceded by a sore throat.

**Examination**

There are areas of thick scale on the scalp, and numerous small, red, scaly lesions on the trunk and limbs (Figure C12.1).

What is the likely diagnosis?

Figure C12.1

## Case study 13

A mother presents with her 13-year-old daughter to her family doctor, because the young girl has recently developed a small isolated patch of hair loss on the back of her scalp. She is otherwise perfectly well.

**Examination**

There is a circumscribed area of hair loss on the occiput. The affected area of scalp is not scaly, and there is no evidence of scarring (Figure C13.1).

What is the most likely diagnosis?

Figure C13.1

## Case study 14

An 18-year-old girl presents with a rash on her chin. Following a diagnosis of mild eczema 3 months previously, she had been applying a topical steroid and an emollient. When the rash did not improve the strength of the topical steroid was increased.

**Examination**

There are numerous papules around her mouth (Figure C14.1).

What is the likely cause of her problem?

Figure C14.1

## Case study 15

A 26-year-old mother of two children presents with her 11-month-old daughter who has lesions on her face and right arm, first noticed 1 week ago. Her 3-year-old son has similar lesions.

**Examination**

There are red, superficially eroded areas with golden crusts on the surface.

What is the diagnosis?

Figure C15.1

# Multiple choice questions

1. **Which of the following are potential adverse effects of potent topical corticosteroids?**

   A   Striae
   B   Hypopituitarism
   C   Tinea incognito
   D   Alopecia
   E   Seborrhoeic keratoses

2. **Which of the following may be associated with pyoderma gangrenosum?**

   A   Cholangiocarcinoma
   B   Monoclonal gammopathy
   C   Regional ileitis
   D   Pancreatic glucagonoma
   E   Rheumatoid arthritis

3. **Erythema multiforme may be triggered by which of the following?**

   A   Herpes simplex
   B   Mycoplasma infection
   C   Orf
   D   Staphylococcal infection
   E   Drugs

4. **The Koebner phenomenon is a feature of which of the following diseases?**

   A   Toxic epidermal necrolysis
   B   Psoriasis
   C   Vitiligo
   D   Atopic dermatitis
   E   Lichen planus

5. **Which of the following can indicate an underlying malignancy?**

   A   Dermatomyositis
   B   Generalized pruritus
   C   Geographic tongue
   D   Acanthosis nigricans
   E   Acquired ichthyosis

6. **Clothing (body) lice are responsible for transmission of which of the following diseases?**

   A   Epidemic typhus
   B   Lyme disease
   C   Bubonic plague
   D   Trypanosomiasis
   E   Malaria

7. **There is a known association between crusted (Norwegian) scabies and which of the following?**

   A   Erythrodermic psoriasis
   B   HIV/AIDS
   C   Down's syndrome
   D   Darier's disease
   E   Ichthyosis

8. **Which of the following are true of scabies?**

   A   Itching develops 4–6 weeks after initial infection
   B   Mites live in the hair follicles
   C   Contact with clothing worn by an infected individual often results in transmission of the disease
   D   Red papules on the penis and scrotum are an important physical sign
   E   A Scandinavian species of *Sarcoptes* is responsible for Norwegian scabies

9. **Which of the following are signs of venous hypertension?**

   A   Ulceration between the toes
   B   Atrophie blanche
   C   Cold feet
   D   Lipodermatosclerosis
   E   Pigmentation of the lower leg

10. **Physical signs in tuberous sclerosis complex include which of the following?**

    A   Periungual fibromas
    B   Crowe's sign
    C   Shagreen patch
    D   Multiple lentigines
    E   Auspitz sign

11. Which of the following are recognized causes of erythema nodosum?

   A   Primary tuberculosis
   B   Rheumatoid arthritis
   C   Ulcerative colitis
   D   Lead poisoning
   E   Typhoid

12. Subepidermal blisters are seen in which of the following?

   A   Porphyria cutanea tarda
   B   Pemphigus foliaceus
   C   Bullous impetigo
   D   Cicatricial pemphigoid
   E   Dermatitis herpetiformis

13. Which of the following are recognized treatments for severe psoriasis?

   A   Methotrexate
   B   BCG vaccination
   C   Capsaicin
   D   Acitretin
   E   Biologic agents

14. The Nikolsky sign is a feature of which of the following diseases?

   A   Toxic epidermal necrolysis
   B   Psoriasis
   C   Vitiligo
   D   Atopic dermatitis
   E   Pemphigus vulgaris

15. Which of the following are cutaneous features of systemic sclerosis?

   A   Calcinosis
   B   Raynaud's phenomenon
   C   Ecchymoses
   D   Gottron's papules
   E   Photosensitivity

16. Onycholysis may be a sign of which of the following?

   A   Thyrotoxicosis
   B   Myxoedema
   C   Calcium deficiency
   D   Lichen planus
   E   Psoriasis

17. Which of the following may lead to exfoliative dermatitis (erythroderma)?

   A   Lead poisoning
   B   Cutaneous T-cell lymphoma
   C   Psoriasis
   D   Scurvy
   E   Drug allergy

18. Nail pits occur in association with which of the following?

   A   Alopecia areata
   B   Cirrhosis
   C   Chronic renal failure
   D   Vitamin D deficiency
   E   Psoriasis

19. Cutaneous vasculitis may be associated with which of the following?

   A   *Trichophyton rubrum* infection
   B   Rheumatoid arthritis
   C   Streptococcal infection
   D   Wegener's granulomatosis
   E   Cryoantibodies

20. Which of the following are recognized treatments for atopic dermatitis?

   A   Isotretinoin
   B   Topical tacrolimus
   C   Desensitization injections
   D   Topical corticosteroids
   E   Interferon-α

# Answers to case study questions

## Case study 1

**Diagnosis**
The scaly lesions are patches of Bowen's disease (squamous cell carcinoma confined to the epidermis). The tumour is an invasive squamous cell carcinoma that has developed on one of these patches.

## Case study 2

**Diagnosis**
This child was thought to have ringworm (tinea) on the dorsum of the foot, hence the topical antifungal treatment. However, this would be an unusual infection in a child, there is no scaling (which would be a feature of tinea), and if this was indeed the diagnosis there would have been a response to antifungals. The diagnosis is granuloma annulare—the dorsa of the hands and feet being typical sites.

## Case study 3

**Diagnosis**
Her past history of childhood eczema and asthma indicates that she is atopic. Although she may not have had any problems with eczema since childhood, she is susceptible not only to a recrudescence of atopic eczema but also to irritant dermatitis, and may develop problems in any occupation in which she is exposed to skin irritants—in hairdressing she is exposed to irritants on a daily basis, e.g. when shampooing clients' hair. She is also exposed to numerous chemicals, including hair dyes, which can cause allergic contact dermatitis. Patch testing will help to establish if she has contact allergy. Work as a hairdresser is contraindicated in anyone with a history of atopy.

## Case study 4

**Diagnosis**
(a) This is psoriasis.
(b) This is eczema. Always consider contact allergy to components of footwear and carry out patch testing.
(c) This is tinea—so-called 'moccasin'-type athlete's foot, because the distribution suggests the shape of a moccasin. The recent development of a rash in the groins suggests that the infection has been spread to this area.

## Case study 5

**Diagnosis**
This is a lentigo maligna. A nodular melanoma may develop within the lentigo. The treatment of choice for lentigo maligna is excision, but if this would be difficult to perform because of the size or site of the lesion radiotherapy is an alternative—the lesion is radiosensitive.

## Case study 6

**Diagnosis**
These are the papular lesions of molluscum contagiosum, which are often numerous in individuals with atopic dermatitis, the background dermatosis in this case. When they resolve in people with atopy they often leave a temporary pitted scar similar to that after a chickenpox lesion.

## Case study 7

**Diagnosis**
This is tinea. The well-defined inflammatory margin separating normal and abnormal skin is typical. Always check other areas of the body that are frequent sites of tinea infection, particularly the feet, because these are invariably involved.

## Case study 8

**Diagnosis**

This is bullous pemphigoid. It often presents as generalized itching that lasts for weeks or months before the blisters appear. It typically affects older people, the blisters are tense because they are subepidermal, and oral blisters are infrequent, unlike pemphigus.

## Case study 9

**Diagnosis**

This is tinea incognito—tinea modified by inappropriate use of potent topical steroids.

The clear-cut marginal erythema is replaced by ill-defined areas of scaling erythema, often studded with inflammatory papules and pustules. Microscopy of scrapings shows an abundance of fungal mycelium. He also has athlete's foot.

## Case study 10

**Diagnosis**

This patient has developed angioedema, probably as a result of hypersensitivity to the ACE (angiotensin-converting enzyme) inhibitor.

You should check that the airway is not compromised, and that the patient is breathing normally and is not hypotensive. The drug should be stopped and treatment initiated with adrenaline. Antihistamines do not work in this type of angioedema.

## Case study 11

**Diagnosis**

The lesion that bled is probably a basal cell carcinoma. The other is a malignant melanoma. The surrounding skin shows evidence of chronic sun damage.

## Case study 12

**Diagnosis**

This is the typical history and appearance of guttate (drop-like) psoriasis. It is characteristically seen in younger patients and often follows a streptococcal infection of the throat.

## Case study 13

**Diagnosis**

The diagnosis is alopecia areata. Reassurance should be given that it is most likely that hair will re-grow in the coming weeks. However, in some cases the hair loss will become more extensive, causing considerable stress and anxiety.

## Case study 14

**Diagnosis**

This is a typical history of perioral dermatitis, in which topical steroid use is thought to be an important causative factor. The patient should stop all topical steroids and take an oral tetracycline or erythromycin for 6–8 weeks.

## Case study 15

**Diagnosis**

This woman's baby has impetigo as, almost certainly, does her son. Treatment is a course of an anti-staphylococcal antibiotic.

# Answers to multiple choice questions

1. A, C
2. B, C, E
3. A, B, C, E
4. B, C, E
5. A, B, D, E
6. A
7. B, C
8. A, D
9. B, D, E
10. A, C
11. A, C
12. A, D, E
13. A, D, E
14. A, E
15. A, B
16. A, E
17. B, C, E
18. A, E
19. B, C, D, E
20. B, D

# Glossary of dermatological terms

abscess: a localized collection of pus in a cavity formed by disintegration or necrosis of tissues, and usually caused by a microorganism.

acantholysis (Gk *akantha*—thorn—and *lyein*—to loosen, free): separation of epidermal keratinocytes resulting from loss of intercellular connections (desmosomes), causing the cells to become rounded and resulting in clefts. As occurs in pemphigus and Darier's disease.

acanthosis (Gk *akantha*—thorn, prickle): increased thickness of the prickle-cell layer of the epidermis. As occurs in psoriasis and lichenified eczema.

acro- (Gk *akros*—outermost, extreme): tip, extremity or top. As in thyrotoxic acropachy.

acrochordon: skin tag.

actinic (Gk *aktis, aktinos*—ray): pertaining to rays or beams of light. As in actinic keratosis.

acuminate (L *acuminatus*—pointed, sharpened): tapering or sharply pointed. As in acuminate warts.

agminate (L *agmen, agminis*—group): grouped lesions.

alopecia (Gk *alōpekia*—a disease similar to the mange of foxes): loss of hair.

angiokeratoma: a vascular lesion in which dilatation of blood vessels is combined with hyperkeratosis.

anhidrosis: lack of sweating.

aphthae: painful ulcers of mucosae.

apocrine: relating to a gland that produces a secretion containing not only fluid but also cellular granules.

aquagenic: caused by contact with water. As in aquagenic pruritus.

arborizing (L *arbor*—tree): branching, as of a tree, e.g. arborizing telangiectasia.

atopy (atopic): predisposing to the development of diseases associated with excessive IgE antibody formation.

atrophy: a wasting or shrinking of a cell, tissue or organ.

Auspitz sign: a sign described by an Austrian dermatologist that features punctate haemorrhage from superficial dermal capillaries upon removal of scale in psoriasis.

balanitis: inflammation of the glans penis.

balanoposthitis: inflammation of the glans penis and prepuce.

balsam of Peru: mixture of oil and resin obtained from the tree *Myroxolon pereirae*. Used as an antiseptic.

Beau's lines: transverse depressions on the nail plates associated with growth arrest during serious illness.

Becker's naevus: hairy, pigmented epidermal naevus occurring on shoulder area.

Behçet's syndrome: named after a Turkish dermatologist; the main features of this syndrome are orogenital ulceration and iritis.

berloque dermatitis (Fr *berloque*—a pendant): a streaky form of pigmented photodermatitis occurring on the neck and caused by psoralens, usually bergamot oil, in perfumes.

Besnier's prurigo: an alternative name for atopic dermatitis.

Blaschko's lines: a system of lines, the pattern of which is followed by many naevoid skin conditions.

blepharitis: inflammation of the eyelid.

boil: colloquial term for a furuncle.

Bowen's disease: epidermal squamous cell carcinoma *in situ*.

bromhidrosis (Gk *bromos*—stench—and *hidrōs*—sweat): foul-smelling sweat, usually resulting from bacterial action on axillary apocrine secretions.

bulla (pl. bullae) (L *bulla*—a bubble): a blister; a fluid-filled bleb.

**burrow:** a tunnel in the epidermis occupied by the scabies mite.

**callus (callosity):** localized thickening of the skin, particularly the horny layer, in response to repeated pressure or friction.

**Campbell de Morgan spots:** cherry angiomas. Small, age-related vascular lesions. Campbell de Morgan was a British physician.

**canities (L *canities*—grey hair):** greying or whitening of hair.

**carbuncle:** a deep infection of a group of contiguous hair follicles with *Staphylococcus aureus*, resulting in the formation of a multiloculated abscess.

**Casal's necklace:** an area of erythema and pigmentation around the neck, occurring in pellagra.

**cheilitis (Gk *cheilos*—lip):** inflammation of the lips.

**cheiro- (Gk *cheiros*—hand):** meaning hand.

**cheiropompholyx:** a blistering eruption of the hands.

**cheloid:** alternative spelling of keloid.

**chilblain:** a lesion resulting from a vascular response to cold. Also called pernio, perniosis.

**chloasma:** patchy pigmentation of the face. Also known as melasma.

**chrysiasis:** deposition of gold in the tissues.

**clavus:** a corn.

**colophony:** rosin obtained from pine trees. Many uses, but perhaps best known as a component of adhesive plasters.

**comedo:** a plug in a pilosebaceous follicle.

**condyloma (pl. condylomata):** wart-like tumour or growth. Usually applied to genital warts (condylomata acuminata) and secondary syphilitic lesions in the anogenital region (condylomata lata).

**conglobata (L *conglobare*—to gather into a rounded form):** clumped or clustered. As used in a severe type of acne (acne conglobata).

**craquelé:** cracked. Resembling crazy paving. As in eczema craquelé.

**Crowe's sign:** axillary freckling in neurofibromatosis.

**CRST (CREST) syndrome:** most common form of systemic sclerosis. **c**alcinosis, **R**aynaud's phenomenon, (o)**e**sophageal involvement, **s**clerodactyly, **t**elangiectasia.

**cyst:** any closed cavity or sac with a lining and containing fluid or other material.

**dandruff:** a popular term for pityriasis capitis.

**Darier's sign:** named after a famous French dermatologist, this is the occurrence of weals on rubbing lesions of urticaria pigmentosa.

**Dennie–Morgan folds:** prominent folds in lower eyelid skin seen in atopic individuals.

**depilation (epilation):** removal of hair.

**depilatory:** any agent used to remove or destroy hair.

**dermabrasion:** removal of skin lesions by a variety of abrading devices such as a rapidly turning wire brush.

**dermatoglyphics:** epidermal ridge patterns on hands and feet.

**dhobi itch:** colloquial term used for any itchy condition affecting the groins/pubic region, particularly ringworm. A dhobi is an Indian washerman.

**diascopy:** examination of a skin lesion by applying firm pressure over it with a glass slide. Used particularly to demonstrate 'apple-jelly' nodules in lupus vulgaris.

**dyschromatosis:** abnormal pigmentation.

**dyskeratosis:** abnormal keratinization.

**dysmorphophobia:** a disturbance in perception of body image.

**ecchymosis:** a bruise

**ectasia:** dilatation of a duct or vessel. As in lymphangiectasia.

**ecthyma:** a heavily crusted, deep-seated, pyogenic infection.

**eczema:** an inflammatory skin reaction characterized by itching, redness, vesiculation, exudation and crusting.

**ephelis:** a freckle.

**epidermotropism:** movement towards the epidermis.

**epiloia:** derived from **epi**lepsy, **lo**w **i**ntelligence and **a**denoma sebaceum. An alternative name for tuberous sclerosis complex.

**erysipelas:** a superficial form of cellulitis caused by haemolytic streptococci.

**erythema (Gk *erythēma*—redness):** redness of the skin.

**furuncle:** localized pyogenic inflammation in a hair follicle. Also known as a boil.

**glabrous:** smooth, hairless skin.

**Gottron's papules:** erythematous papules overlying finger joints in dermatomyositis.

**Hansen's disease:** leprosy. Hansen was a Norwegian bacteriologist who first demonstrated *Mycobacterium leprae*.

**herpetiform:** grouped vesicles resembling herpes.

**hirsutism (L *hirsutus*—shaggy):** the growth of hair in women in the male sexual pattern.

**hives:** popular US term for urticaria.

**ichthyosis (Gk *ichthys*—fish):** a group of disorders of keratinization characterized by scaling likened to fish skin.

**intertrigo:** nflammation of apposed skin surfaces such as groins, axillae and inframammary regions.

**Kaposi's varicelliform eruption:** named after a famous Hungarian-born dermatologist, this is disseminated infection with herpes simplex or vaccinia virus in atopic individuals.

**keloid (cheloid):** excessive scar tissue formation extending beyond the original area of injury.

**kerion (GK *kērion*—honeycomb):** a severe inflammatory response to the presence of fungal infection, usually of animal origin, on hair-bearing areas.

**Koebner (Köbner) phenomenon:** the provocation of skin lesions by trauma, seen in psoriasis, lichen planus and vitiligo. Köbner was a German dermatologist.

**Koenen's tumours:** periungual fibromas in tuberous sclerosis complex.

**koilonychia (Gk *koilos*—hollow—and *onychos*—nail):** spoon-shaped nails, typically a feature of severe iron deficiency.

**Langerhans' cells:** epidermal dendritic cells, characterized by the presence of racquet-shaped 'Birbeck' granules, acting as specialized antigen-presenting cells.

**Lassar's paste:** zinc oxide paste with salicylic acid.

**lentigo:** a pigmented macule with an increased number of melanocytes at the dermoepidermal junction.

**leukoderma (leucoderma) (Gk *leukos*—white—and *derma*—skin):** lack of normal pigmentation of the skin. Non-specific term that in lay usage is often applied to vitiligo.

**leukoplakia:** persistent white patches on mucous membranes.

**lichen (Gk *leichēn*—a tree moss):** resembling a tree moss/lichen. As in lichen planus.

**lichenification:** thickening and coarsening of the skin, associated with rubbing and scratching (e.g. in atopic eczema).

**lichenoid:** resembling lichen planus.

**livedo (L *livere*—to be blue or bluish):** a cyanotic discoloration of the skin that follows the cutaneous vascular network.

**lupus (L *lupus*—wolf):** applied to lesions that involve tissue damage likened to the gnawing of a wolf, e.g. lupus vulgaris and lupus erythematosus.

**Lyell's syndrome:** toxic epidermal necrolysis.

**Lyme disease:** Lyme is a town in Connecticut where the association between ticks, a spirochaete (*Borrelia burgdorferi*), and an arthropathy was first established.

**madarosis:** loss of eyelashes.

**Madura foot:** named after a town in southern India, it is another name for a mycetoma.

**Mees' lines:** transverse white bands on the nails in arsenic and thallium poisoning.

**melasma:** patchy hyperpigmentation of the face. Also known as chloasma.

**milium (pl. milia) (L *milium*—millet seed):** tiny white keratin cyst.

**Mohs' micrographic surgery:** Named after the US surgeon who developed the technique, this is a method of layer-by-layer excision of tumours with histological assessment of excision margins.

**morbilliform:** measles-like.

**Muehrke's striae:** white bands on the nail occurring in severe hypoalbuminaemia.

**myiasis (Gk *myia*—a fly):** invasion of tissues by fly larvae.

**naevus:** a localized cutaneous malformation involving either an excess or relative deficiency of any of the normal cutaneous structures. A cutaneous hamartoma.

**necrobiosis:** physiological or normal cell death in the midst of living tissue. As in necrobiosis lipoidica.

necrolysis (Gk *nekros*—dead—and *lyein* to loosen, free): separation of dead tissue. As in the epidermis in toxic epidermal necrolysis.

Nikolsky's sign: separation of the epidermis produced by firm sliding pressure of the finger. Occurs in pemphigus and toxic epidermal necrolysis. Nikolsky was a Russian dermatologist.

nitidus: glistening, shiny. As in lichen nitidus.

nummular (L *nummulus* dim. of *nummus*—coin): in the shape of a coin. Discoid.

onychogryphosis (Gk *onychos*—nail—and *grypos*—curved, hooked): thickening and overcurvature of the nail resembling a ram's horn.

onychoschizia (Gk *onychos*—nail—and *schizein*—to cleave or split): splitting of the nail plate into layers.

ophiasis (Gk *ophis*—snake): snake-like. A pattern of alopecia areata affecting the scalp margin.

pachyonychia (Gk *pachys*—thick—and *onychos*—nail): abnormally thick nails.

papilloma: a nipple-like projection from the skin.

Pautrier's abscess: focal collection of lymphocytes in the epidermis in mycosis fungoides.

peau d'orange: a dimpling appearance of the skin simulating orange peel. Seen in carcinoma of the breast.

pellagra: a disorder caused by dietary deficiency of niacin (nicotinic acid).

perléche (Fr *pourlécher*—to lick all over): angular cheilitis.

pernio (perniosis) (L *pernio*—chilblain): chilblain.

petechia (pl. petechiae): a punctate haemorrhagic spot.

photo- (Gk *phōtos*—light): pertaining to light.

phyto- (Gk *phyton*—plant, tree): pertaining to plants.

pityriasis (L *pityriasis*—scurf, from Gk *pityron*—bran): a branny scaling of the skin. As in pityriasis versicolor.

poikiloderma (Gk *poikilos*—mottled, dappled—and *derma*—skin): dappled pigmentation, usually associated with telangiectasia and atrophy.

poliosis (Gk *poliosis*—becoming grey): localized patches of white hair. As in piebaldism.

pompholyx (Gk *pompholyx*—a bubble): acute vesiculobullous eruption on hands (cheiro-) and feet (podo-).

prurigo (L *prurigo*—itching): term used in some conditions associated with itching, including nodular prurigo and Besnier's prurigo (atopic dermatitis).

psoriasiform: resembling psoriasis.

psoriasis (Gk *psōriasis, psōra*—itch, mange, scab): a chronic skin disease typically manifesting scaly plaques.

pterygium (Gk *pterygion*—wing): used to denote a web or fold of skin, e.g. pterygium colli (webbed neck in Turner's syndrome) and the tissue encroaching on the nail apparatus in lichen planus of the nails.

pyoderma: generic name for any purulent skin condition.

reticulate (L *reticulatus*—net-shaped): in a net-like pattern.

rhinophyma (Gk *rhis, rhinos*—nose—and *phyma*—inflamed swelling): connective tissue and sebaceous gland hypertrophy of the nose as a feature of rosacea in men.

sclerosis (Gk *sklēros*—hard): thickening, induration.

shagreen (Fr *peau de chagrin*): resembling shark skin or untanned leather with a rough surface. As in shagreen patches—connective tissue naevi on the back in tuberous sclerosis complex.

shingles (L *cingulum*—girdle, belt): colloquial term for herpes zoster.

Sister Joseph's nodule: umbilical metastasis from intra-abdominal neoplasm. Named after Sister Mary Joseph who worked with Dr William James Mayo and is said to have pointed out its significance to him.

squame (L *squama*—a scale of a fish or serpent): a scale.

sycosis (Gk *sykon*—a fig): deep inflammation of hair follicles. As in sycosis barbae—inflammation of the beard area.

telangiectasia (telangiectasis) (Gk *telos*—end, *angeion*—vessel—and *ektasis*—dilatation): dilatation of small blood vessels.

tinea (L *tinea*—a gnawing worm): a dermatophyte fungal infection.

trich-, tricho- (Gk *trichos*—hair): relating to hair. As in trichology.

trichotillomania: compulsive hair pulling.

trichophytid: a rash provoked by an immunological response to a fungal infection, e.g. pompholyx on the hands provoked by a severe inflammatory fungal infection on the foot.

verruca: in common use referring to a plantar wart, but in fact a term applicable to a wart at any site.

weal: this is the correct spelling. A transient, raised, itchy lesion occurring in urticaria and dermographism.

whitlow: infection of finger pulp. As in herpetic whitlow.

Wickham's striae: pattern of lace-like greyish-white lines on the surface of lesions of lichen planus. Louis Wickham was a French dermatologist.

Wood's light: a source of filtered ultraviolet light that is used to demonstrate fluorescence caused by certain organisms, e.g. *Microsporum canis* [tinea capitis] (yellow–green) and *Corynebacterium minutissimum* [erythrasma] (coral pink).

xerosis (Gk *xeros*—dry): dryness.

# Index

Page numbers in *italics* indicate illustrations that are not on the same page as the relevant text.